Vivid Living

7 Powerful Health Hacks to Restore Your Body &
Achieve Vibrant Health in Just 10 Minutes a Day

Refresh | Recharge | Nourish | Rebuild | Detoxify | Revitalize | Unleash

D1455281

Alex Bradford

Praise for Vivid Living

"There is so much content and information on the internet about healthy living, I always felt overwhelmed and never knew where to start. Vivid Living's 7-day course makes it easy and simple to actually put these proven tips to work in your daily life and START creating a healthier lifestyle right away. It covers important topics regarding your overall wellness, and I even find myself constantly referring to it for reminders! I especially love the 10-minute workout bonus... How can you argue with setting aside only 10 minutes a day? Vivid Living's 7-day course is worth every penny!

Lauren M.
Texas, USA

"Vivid Living changed so many things for me. While I loved many aspects of the program, I have to say that one stands out as the most pivotal. The sections on how to stop and properly nourish my body followed by how to easily revitalize my spirit - with practical tools on how to do it - made it possible for me to keep going with the other courses.

I'm hard on myself. I push myself to ridiculous lengths. I give myself no quarter when it comes to sleep, breathing, and remembering that nothing I strive for means anything if I'm exhausted or sick.

Some of the lessons I used as they were and others I tweaked to fit my personality and routine. All of them made an impact and I'm so glad I took the leap of faith when my friend Alex said, "You need to do this. You need it for your body, mind, and spirit."

She was right. I feel rejuvenated and ready to focus on the things I work so hard for every day. I feel clearer and cleaner than I have in years.

I say the same thing to you...you need to do this. You need it for your body, mind, and spirit.

Shayne McClendon
Amazon Best Selling Author

Contents

INTRODUCTION

I want to thank and congratulate you for choosing Vivid Living. Before you dive into this book, I'd like you to remember **one tiny concept:**

Simple changes over time create a healthier you.

Your health is more than just a blood pressure reading! It's composed of physical, emotional, and spiritual aspects. To improve your *physical* health, you need to engage your *mind*, your *body*, and your *spirit*.

No matter where you're starting on your personal journey to better health, taking the first step is the most difficult and fear-inducing.

Often we don't take action – not because we're afraid of change – but because we're too overwhelmed and don't know where to begin.

The key to Vivid Living is that each action step is broken down into an easy, science-based life-hack or habit that you can start today.

You don't need to think about anything else. You simply take one action step starting now.

I have to mention one small caveat. Vivid Living comes with five easy-to-make delicious dinners. I recommend you bring this book with you shopping.

Take the time to go grocery shopping first. Then you can cook your first meal tonight and take the time to enjoy it. It's going to be delightful. I guarantee it.

What truly matters is you've made the decision to take one positive action step towards improving your health and well-being.

Don't tell yourself, "I'm too busy."

If you want to live a long and healthy life, you have to take care of your most important asset – that's YOU!

After all, it's consistent **habits** that matter most. Let's say you found your "motivation" and decided you were going to work out at the gym hard for two hours. I mean a really hard workout...like lifting small cars and doing 80 pushups in a row, kind of hard.

Then you stop for six months. For six months, you sit on your couch and do nothing. One day, you decide you're going to work out at the gym for two hours again.

What do you think you're accomplishing with a plan like this?

Nothing. That's right...nothing. Working out once every six months like a lunatic isn't going to do anything for your long-term health and longevity.

However, if you **commit to spending just 10 minutes a day to transform yourself** – taking in all aspects of health (mental, emotional, and physical), in a matter of days or weeks, you're going to see and feel dramatic improvements in your overall wellbeing.

Don't fall into the trap that carving out 10 minutes a day for YOURSELF is *difficult*. **It's not.** Beating cancer is HARD. Losing 100 pounds is TOUGH. Quitting smoking is CHALLENGING. Losing a loved one is HEART BREAKING.

This task is easy. You can do this.

More importantly, **you need to need to do this**. This is vitally important if you're feeling achy, sick, sluggish, or just plain run-down in any area of your life.

With each passing year, you want to have *more* energy and vibrancy. After all, life really starts to get good at 40...so you don't want to reach your

60's, 70's, 80's, or 90's feeling as if you barely have the energy to stay awake.

You deserve so much more.

That's why I'm here to help you on the journey you've chosen to take. I welcome you to Vivid Living, and honor you for making this important decision. I applaud you.

You've chosen to take the time to care for the only true place you'll ever have to live as you travel this glorious, inspiring, and sometimes challenging world.

Be vivid. Be vibrant.

Most of all, live everyday with full intention and make the choices that are going to benefit your health and wellbeing first. *Everything else comes second.*

If you can't help yourself then how can you possibly help anyone else?

10 minutes is all it takes.

Of course, there's one exception. The dinners I've included in the book will take slightly longer than ten minutes to make. :) I'm sure you'll enjoy every delicious mouth-watering bite, so it's definitely worth your time.

In the next few minutes, you'll discover simple, scientifically proven steps to extend your life, shield your body from disease, and increase your wellness and vitality!

It all starts right now!

Once you implement these simple yet effective habits or bio-hacks, you'll restore your vitality, become stronger, feel amazing, look better, and even live longer.

I'm going to ease you into better health in just 10 minutes a day. Day one is going to be so refreshing...you'll wonder why you didn't put these habits in place sooner. That's okay! You're starting now and you're going to be amazing.

Are you ready? Great! Let's get started with your first day of vivid living!

GROCERY LIST

By reviewing the **Vivid Living Shopping List** in advance, you can shop and then pre-plan when you want to cook your delicious superfood dinners.

That's incredibly important!

I want you to have a nourishing dinner every night. Please plan accordingly and take the time to go grocery shopping, so you can get the maximum benefit from Vivid Living.

MEATS / POULTRY / SEAFOOD

- ☐ bacon
- ☐ grass fed ground beef
- ☐ lamb chops
- ☐ peeled wild shrimp
- ☐ whitefish or other seafood

STARCHES

- ☐ beluga lentils
- ☐ naan bread
- ☐ raw quinoa
- ☐ yukon gold or red bliss potatoes *Optional

VEGETABLES / HERBS

- ☐ fresh tomatoes or canned chopped tomatoes (bpa-free)
- ☐ beet greens with roots
- ☐ cabbage (Napa, Savoy, green, or red)
- ☐ carrots
- ☐ cauliflower
- ☐ celery
- ☐ cremini mushrooms
- ☐ dried figs
- ☐ fresh Italian parsley
- ☐ grapefruit
- ☐ green bell pepper
- ☐ green chili pepper or jalapeno
- ☐ parsnips
- ☐ red bell pepper
- ☐ red onions
- ☐ scallions
- ☐ shiitake mushrooms
- ☐ Swiss chard
- ☐ turnips
- ☐ watercress
- ☐ yellow onions

GROCERY LIST

FRUITS
- ☐ lemon
- ☐ limes
- ☐ mango

DAIRY
- ☐ grass-fed butter
- ☐ feta
- ☐ full fat Greek yogurt
- ☐ heavy cream *Optional*
- ☐ ghee

ESSENTIALS
- ☐ apple cider vinegar
- ☐ cayenne chili pepper or red chili pepper
- ☐ chinkiang vinegar *Optional*
- ☐ coconut aminos *Optional*
- ☐ extra virgin coconut oil
- ☐ extra virgin olive oil
- ☐ full fat organic coconut milk
- ☐ old fashioned rolled oats
- ☐ organic chicken stock
- ☐ red wine vinegar
- ☐ rice vinegar
- ☐ sesame oil
- ☐ soy sauce
- ☐ sugar in the raw
- ☐ tamari *Optional*
- ☐ tomato paste

SPICES
- ☐ allspice
- ☐ bay leaf
- ☐ black pepper
- ☐ brown sugar
- ☐ cardamom
- ☐ cayenne pepper
- ☐ clove
- ☐ coriander
- ☐ cumin
- ☐ curry powder
- ☐ fresh ginger
- ☐ garlic
- ☐ garlic powder
- ☐ ginger
- ☐ nutmeg
- ☐ onion powder
- ☐ oregano
- ☐ paprika
- ☐ red pepper flakes
- ☐ rosemary - fresh
- ☐ sage - fresh
- ☐ sea salt
- ☐ sesame seeds - white and black
- ☐ turmeric

Day 1
REFRESH

GET READY TO BE REFRESHED AND REVITALIZED!

Welcome to Vivid Living! Today is your first day to better health!

Drink Up & Then Drink Some More...Why You Need Lemon Water

This topic may seem like a no-brainer, but stick with me here. You'll be guzzling lemon water by the gallon when you realize how this one small change can truly affect your health.

Did you know your body is 75% water?

We are literally more water than anything else, yet we don't give this life-sustaining fluid enough credit for our health and well-being.

Water makes up approximately 75% of your muscles and brain. It's 83% of your blood and 22% of your bones. Water helps your body absorb nutrients. It also removes waste, protects and cushions vital organs and joints, moistens oxygen for breathing, and helps convert food into energy.

After a long day, when you finally lay your head on that fluffy pillow, your brain is resting and your body is being rebuilt overnight. As you sleep, your hormones are balanced, energy is restored, body tissues grow and are repaired, your blood pressure drops, and your body temperature drops.

When you wake up, you've lost weight through exhalation of water vapor. Your tissues are partially dehydrated and your body has eliminated numerous internal toxins.

Every day, you wake up water and carbon-depleted and about three pounds (1.5kg) lighter than before you fell asleep. **Your body is thirsty. It will thank you if you start every day with a simple glass of lemon water.**

By squeezing freshly cut lemon into a glass of distilled water at room temperature, you fuel up with electrolytes.

Lemons contain potassium, calcium, and magnesium for electrolyte replenishment.

Note: **Distilled water** is the closest you can get to pure water and it is my number

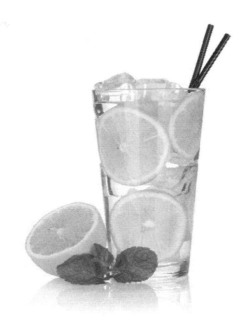

one pick. You can also boil or filter your water to remove toxins and impurities. **Spring water** is also fine to use.

Lemon water isn't just great for the morning. If you've finished an intense workout, hot yoga, or even a leisurely walk – lemon water is a great way quench your thirst and restore your vitality.

I urge you to sip lemon water throughout the day. Your cells are going to do a happy dance.

If you feel dehydrated, don't reach for Gatorade or other popular sports drinks! One of the worst ingredients found in Gatorade is "brominated vegetable oil," added to prevent it from becoming cloudy and to keep the artificial flavorings suspended in the liquid. The effect of these added chemical toxins far outweigh the minimal benefits you might get from drinking it.

If you prefer a hot beverage when you wake-up, you can add fresh lemon to warm water.

Since lemon contains citric acid, it interacts with other enzymes and acids to help stimulate digestion and jumpstart liver enzymes.

Lemons also contain high amounts of vitamin C – something your body needs to manufacture glutathione. Also known as the "mother of all anti-oxidants," glutathione is used to **neutralize toxins and detoxify the liver**. The vitamin C in lemon is a powerful antioxidant in its own right. It helps rejuvenate the look and feel of your skin while increasing the speed of wound healing.

One of the great nutritional qualities of lemons is the benefit to your liver. According to Dr. Alexander F. Beddoe in *Biological Ionization in Human Nutrition*, **the liver can make more enzymes out of fresh lemon juice than any other food element**.

Given more of the raw materials needed to function properly, the **liver's efficiency gets a boost** from lemon consumption.

As published by Dutch researchers in a 2002 edition of the *European Journal of Nutrition*, lemon peels and the waste stream of the lemon peels are effective in lowering blood and liver cholesterol levels. Although performed on animal subjects, these results suggest that lemon peel consumption could be **beneficial to people with fatty liver disease**.

Water with lemon is also a great **anti-inflammatory food**. If you feel a sore throat coming on or are prone to respiratory tract infections, lemon water can help soothe your throat and relieve inflammation.

Your nervous system needs a significant amount of potassium to function properly. The abundant potassium content in lemons can help to **calm your nerves and lower blood pressure** by as much as 10%.

Lemon water can even help you shed fat.

According to 240th National Meeting of the American Chemical Society (ACS) 2010 study, drinking just two eight-ounce cups of water before meals helped dieters lose an extra 5 pounds yearly. That's less water each day than you find in an average bottled beverage...to lose 5 pounds a year! For such a small change, that's a big deal.

Brenda Davy, Ph.D., senior author on the study said, "We found in earlier studies that middle aged and older people who drank two cups of water right before eating a meal ate between **75 and 90 fewer calories during that meal.** In this recent study, we found that over the course of 12 weeks, dieters who drank water before meals, three times per day, lost about 5 pounds more than dieters who did not increase their water intake."

In other words, combine water with lemon for a quick, no-prescription weight loss elixir!

When your body is hydrated, it's easier to lose weight at a greater speed than when it is not.

Recommended Ounces of Water Daily Based on Weight	
100 pounds	67 ounces
110 pounds	74 ounces
120 pounds	80 ounces
130 pounds	87 ounces
140 pounds	94 ounces
150 pounds	100 ounces
160 pounds	107 ounces
170 pounds	114 ounces
180 pounds	121 ounces
190 pounds	127 ounces
200 pounds	134 ounces
210 pounds	141 ounces
220 pounds	148 ounces
230 pounds	154 ounces
240 pounds	161 ounces
250 pounds	168 ounces

Squeeze the juice of one whole lemon into your water and drink up!

(Note: If you currently weigh less than 150 pounds, reduce the juice to half a lemon.)

Mix it up, drink it quickly, and wait half an hour before eating to let your body absorb the maximum benefits of restorative lemon water.

After drinking, rinse your mouth with plain purified water to minimize the wear and tear on your tooth enamel.

The amount of water you should drink daily is based on your weight. A simple guideline is to multiply your weight by 2/3, or 67% (.67). The resulting number is how many ounces of water your body needs to be fully hydrated.

It may seem challenging at first but you can do it. One easy way to drink more lemon water is to use a special container that is only used for your water.

I like (and use) a 24-ounce Tervis Tumbler for my daily water intake. They're BPA-free, virtually indestructible, customizable, and simply great to look at.

Check out the chart above to get the recommended ounces of water that you should drink based on your weight.

Try breaking up your daily water intake as follows:

1. Drink 16 ounces when you wake up
2. Drink 16 ounces before each meal (a total of 48 ounces)
3. Drink 16 ounces before bed

That's 80 ounces for the day (and well on the way to better health)! You can easily increase your water consumption by using a 24-ounce tumbler of water instead of a 16-ounce glass. That will boost your water intake to 120 ounces!

Now that you have your refreshing lemon water, sip away and revel in the benefits that this simple act will have on your health.

Your only homework today is to drink your lemon water. So easy and important to every cell in your body.

Tomorrow is day two! I'll share how to recharge your health with a simple pose...

DAY ONE DINNER

PARSNIP SOUP & GRASS FED MEATLOAF WITH WATERCRESS AND CARROTS

Superfood #1 – Watercress:

Most people are familiar with its popular cousins – broccoli, cabbage, and arugula – and you might have noticed watercress in gourmet salad mixes.

It's been around since the beginning of time. Even Hippocrates built his first hospital close to a stream for a steady supply of the water-growing green.

The leaves are tender and the stalks are crisp, making it a perfect addition to salads, soups, and sandwiches. This slightly peppery leaf veggie is under-appreciated and underrepresented.

Since watercress earned the top spot on the superfood powerhouse list, I decided it deserved top billing.

Watercress is a potent anti-cancer vegetable. It contains high levels of phenyl ethyl isothiocyanate (PEITC) compounds that give this tasty green a serious disease-fighting punch.

Breast, lung, colorectal, and prostate cancer cells are suppressed by the activity of PEITC. This rarely talked about compound works by cutting off the damaged cell's ability to signal your body to make new blood vessels. This is a process known as anti-angiogenesis.

Without the ability to tell your body to create new blood vessels to supply the tumor, the cancer receives no oxygen or nutrition – essentially starving the damaged cancer cells until they die.

Another compound called gluconasturtiin is the source of the slightly peppery taste of watercress and it suppresses carcinogens that lead to cancer. So enjoy this recipe and know that you are helping your body prevent cancer with each delicious bite.

Parsnip Soup Recipe

Serves 4 / Prep Time: 45 minutes / Cook Time: 60 minutes

Ingredients

- 12 ounces parsnips, peeled and cut into 1/2 inch pieces
- 2 carrots, peeled and cut into 1/2-inch pieces
- 2 tablespoon olive oil
- Sea salt and ground black pepper to taste
- ½ of a large onion, diced
- 2 stalks celery, diced
- 1-¼ teaspoons butter
- 2 cloves garlic, minced
- 1 teaspoon brown sugar
- ½ teaspoon ground ginger
- ¼ teaspoon ground cardamom
- ¼ teaspoon ground allspice
- ¼ teaspoon ground nutmeg
- ¼ teaspoon cayenne pepper
- 14 ounces all natural chicken stock
- ½ cup organic coconut milk
- 3 tablespoons heavy cream (or use coconut cream)

Method

1. Preheat oven to 425 degrees F.

2. Place parsnips and carrots into a mixing bowl, sprinkle with 1 table-spoon olive oil. Toss to coat vegetables with oil. Season to taste with salt and pepper. Spread vegetables evenly over baking sheet. Roast until parsnips are tender and golden brown, about 30 minutes.

3. Heat remaining 1 tablespoon olive oil in a large saucepan over medium heat. Stir in onion and celery.

4. Cook and stir until vegetables have softened and onion is beginning to turn golden brown, about 7 minutes. Reduce heat to low. Stir in butter, garlic, brown sugar, and roasted parsnips and carrots. Continue to cook and stir until all vegetables are very tender and beginning to brown, about 10 minutes.

5. Season with ginger, cardamom, allspice, nutmeg, and cayenne pepper; stir for 1 minute. Pour in chicken stock. Bring to a boil over medium-high heat. Reduce heat to medium-low, partially cover, and simmer gently until all vegetables are very tender, about 15 minutes.

6. Pour soup into a blender, filling the pitcher no more than halfway full. Hold down the lid of the blender with a folded kitchen towel. Carefully start the blender, using a few quick pulses to get soup moving before setting to puree. Puree in batches until smooth and pour into a clean pot. Alternately, you can use a stick blender and puree the soup right in the cooking pot.

7. Stir in milk and cream. Return to a simmer over medium-low heat. Season to taste with salt and pepper before serving.

Grass Fed Meatloaf with Watercress and Carrots

Serves 4 / Prep Time: 45 minutes / Cook Time: 60 minutes

Ingredients

- ½ onion chopped
- 2 cloves garlic, minced
- 2 cups watercress, chopped
- ¼ cup chopped green bell pepper
- ¼ cup of grated carrot
- 2 eggs, beaten
- ½ cup of milk
- 2 teaspoons of salt
- ½ teaspoon black pepper
- ½ teaspoon of garlic powder
- ½ teaspoon of onion powder
- ½ teaspoon of paprika
- 1 ½ pounds of grass-fed ground beef (or 1 pound beef with ½ pound pork)
- 1 ½ cups of old-fashioned rolled oats (blended till fine powder)
- 2 tablespoons of tomato paste (plus 1 tablespoon. for the top)

Method

1. Heat oven to 350 degrees F.

2. Sauté onion, garlic, green pepper, water cress, and carrot in coconut oil over medium heat for a couple minutes.

3. Combine beaten eggs with milk, salt, black pepper, garlic powder, and onion powder in a medium bowl.

4. Mix oats into ground meat with your hands. Add egg and milk mixture, sautéed veggies, 2 tablespoons of tomato paste, and mix using your hands.

5. Press the mixture into a meat loaf pan (the kind of pan with drainage holes in the bottom) or a large loaf pan. Bake for 30 minutes. Spread 1 tablespoon of tomato paste mixed with a teaspoon of water and a sprinkle of onion powder over the top of the meatloaf and bake for another hour.

6. Let it sit approximately 10 minutes after removal from oven before slicing to serve.

Day 2
RECHARGE

POWER POSES THAT RECHARGE YOUR HEALTH AND INCREASE CONFIDENCE

Hello my favorite Vivid Lifers...did you do your homework from yesterday? Did you drink your lemon water? *I hope so.*

I really think you're going to love this step to better health. I do this every evening before bed to get the full benefit.

The beauty of Vivid Living is that you can do it whenever you want – the time most convenient for you. The only request I have is that you ACTUALLY take the 10 minutes today and complete this unit.

Remember...*if you aren't functioning at your full health and vitality, how can you be of service to the loved ones around you?*

I want to talk to you about inversions.

If you've never practiced yoga, you might not have heard about inversions. An inversion is simply a pose that reverses the aging force of gravity.

Gravity controls our neurons, bones, muscles, and even the speed at which we age. In space, your muscles would atrophy due to the loss of muscle protein. This effect would contribute to an acceleration in aging. The same effects are found in cases of prolonged bed rest.

Gravity affects aging.

Dr. J. Patrick Meehan, MD, PhD, director of the Human Centrifuge Lab at the University of Southern California School of Medicine since 1954, NASA consultant, and an authority on gravity's effects on the cardiovascular system, says inversion exercises are not dangerous.

The cerebral cage (your skull) protects blood vessels from bursting. In fact, you could be exposed to negative 15g of force without rupture.

With a yoga pose as simple as **Viparita Karani (also known as Legs Up the Wall)** there's no cause for concern. There is only your good health to gain.

Viparita Karani lowers diastolic blood pressure and relieves pressure from the venous return or varicose veins. If you suffer from edema (swelling) of the legs, this pose will relieve pressure by reversing blood and fluid pooling from the day spent standing or sitting.

This position also allows for lymphatic system drainage and helps lymph fluid move towards the heart where it can merge again with vascular system blood and increase the rate at which your lymph system detoxifies your body. By assisting with lymphatic drainage, many symptoms such as fluid retention, varicose veins, and even cellulite tend to be reduced over time.

Another benefit of Viparita Karani is that your heart has to pump harder to get the blood back up to the legs. That makes this a two-for-one exercise. Your mind is resting while your body is working out. It also gives your adrenal glands a chance to rest and reset so they can work together more efficiently with your thyroid.

A little-known fact about Viparita Karani is that it helps balance your hormones. That means that whether you are a man or a woman in the middle of your life, this particular exercise allows your pituitary, thyroid, adrenals, ovaries (in childbearing women), and the pancreas (in men and menopausal women) to clearly and effectively communicate with each other.

Then there's the stress factor. Stress literally makes you lose your mind! When you're under chronic stress, you can't think clearly and you don't make smart decisions. The additional relaxation effect of this yoga pose helps you to relieve some of your daily mental stress. Remaining calm and rational helps get you through your busy day.

When your body works at full speed and efficiency, you feel more secure, grounded, and able to make the best decisions for your life starting now.

Here's how Viparita Karani helps you relax in a matter of minutes!

Before you get started, you'll need:

- Yoga mat

- Yoga bolster, two small blankets, or standard bath towels

- Gently lit room

- Vivid Living Relaxing Classical Music for Busy People Playlist on You-Tube

- Vivid Living Relaxing Ambient Music for Busy People Playlist on You-Tube

If it's your first time doing this pose, you may be a little stiff. The more you do it, the easier it gets…so don't give up!

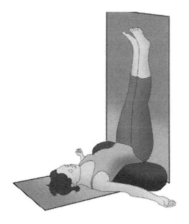

Viparita Karani with support

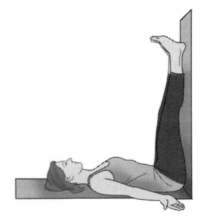

Viparita Karani without support

This pose works to stretch out your hamstrings. If you sit at a desk all day, your hamstrings are going to feel the effects of this pose the most. Power through any light soreness because it lessens over time!

1. Use two thick folded towels, blankets, or a firm round bolster. Place your support about 5 inches away from the wall. If you're stiff, place the support further from the wall. If you're flexible, increase the height of the support.

2. Sit sideways on the right end of the support, with your right side against the wall. Play around with the level of support until it feels right for you. (If you're left-handed you can switch this around.)

3. Now lie down and exhale. Swing your legs up onto the wall. The support should be under your 'sitting bones.' If you slide off your support, adjust it until you're comfortable.

4. Your sitting bones should be close to the wall but they don't need to be right next to it (they don't have to touch the wall). Your upper back should be flat but your lower back should be gently arched.

5. Lift and release your neck to release any tension.

6. Open and separate your shoulder blades by stretching your arms either halfway or all the way out from your sides. Keep your palms facing up.

7. Keep your legs firmly against the wall. If the back of your legs feels tight, bend your knees slightly and slowly straighten them again. Repeat this step until you feel comfortable in the position.

8. Relax your facial muscles, close your eyes, and breathe in and out deeply.

9. Stay in *Legs Up the Wall* or *Viparita Karani* for 5 to 15 minutes.

Practice this technique every day until it feels natural. This is your meditation and relaxation time. The best time is before you go to bed. However, if you have a stressful job or daily life, you might reap more benefit by doing it in the morning before facing your day.

Doing this simple inversion can **elevate your mood, release muscle tension** by up to 35%, and **improve the quality of your sleep**. It improves blood flow to your face, hair, and brain. That means more efficient delivery of crucial nutrients and oxygen.

Viparita Karani will help you think clearly, look more radiant, love your body, and feel more vivid every day.

Bonus: Power Poses That Increase Confidence & Boost Testosterone

Have you ever heard the saying, "Fake it until you make it?" There's a lot of truth to this statement!

By adopting a pose that increases confidence, your body feels more dominant and powerful – and here's the sneaky fun part – your brain catches on to what you're doing!

It responds by providing a hormonal boost in testosterone (the dominance hormone) and lowering cortisol (the stress hormone).

These poses are called **power poses** because they empower your physical self through specific body postures.

Assuming one of these positions when you feel weak, afraid, or unsure of yourself will help on multiple fronts. Primarily, your level of confidence soars and your body becomes more relaxed.

A 2012 Harvard study called *The Benefit of Power Posing before a High Stakes Social Evaluation,* confirmed these findings. If you're preparing for a job interview, a negotiation, a big meeting, or even making a major purchase – these poses can help you achieve the outcome you desire.

Think about how many times you've sat in your chair, shrunk down, trying to make yourself as small as physically possible. How about the last time you were on the phone...did you hunch over in your chair? When you stood up...did you cross your arms over your chest and turn your feet inward?

These nonverbal poses send a signal to your brain that you are powerless. *Worse, they also tell the people around you that you are lacking in power.*

By standing tall and expansive, you convey high power and confidence. Your physical pose is hormonally transmitted to your mind and body. After a power pose you'll feel more positive, in control, and optimistic about your future.

The Columbia University Graduate School of Business studied power posing and found that these positions worked with both male and female participants. They create positive changes in how your neurons release messages to your hormones.

These neuroendocrine communications go beyond mere *thinking* and *feeling*. **They actually affect your physiology and behaviors.**

Power poses help you become goal-oriented and more likely to take action. Here are three poses you'll want to practice for one minute each before your next meeting or high stakes interaction.

POWER POSE #1
The Rocky V

Remember when Rocky Balboa raised both arms over his head in victory and accomplishment? This display is recognized throughout the world as the sign of a winner.

It elevates your mind and increases testosterone levels in your body.

Raise your hands to create a 'V' and hold that pose for 60 seconds. While holding, tell yourself, "**I'm powerful and I** will be **victorious.**"

POWER POSE #2
The Wonder Woman

This stance is iconic. Wonder Woman stood proudly with her hands on her hips. The outward pointing elbows and firmly planted feet make you appear significantly bigger, signal higher authority, and boosts confidence. Hold this pose for 60 seconds.

Say to yourself, "**I'm an authority on this subject** (fill in the blank for you**). I will get the outcome I desire.**"

POWER POSE #3
The Eagle

You can do this pose while sitting. Simply take both your hands, interlace them loosely behind your head, lean back in your chair, and take up as much space as possible.

Hold for 60 seconds and *smile*. Say to yourself, **"I'm proud and grateful for what I will accomplish today."**

Get Posing!

Power pose before your next big moment or life event and your brain will have *no choice* but to make you feel like the winner your body has already communicated that you are!

Congratulations my Vivid Lifer, you've completed day two! Wasn't that easy?

DAY TWO DINNER

CHERMOULA BROILED WHITEFISH & CREAMY ANTI-CANCER VEGGIE CURRY

Superfood #2 – Red Bell Peppers:

Bell peppers originated in Central and South America with seeds of a wild variety dating all the way back to 5000 B.C. Bell peppers earned their place in history when Columbus introduced them to the Old World. He was looking for the valuable black peppercorn and instead he found the bell pepper growing in the West Indies.

The colors and nutritional punch of bell peppers depend on when they are harvested. Green bell peppers are unripe. Yellow and orange are riper and slightly fruity. It's the red bell pepper that's the true star of the show with its sweet floral complexity.

Red bell peppers contain heart saving vitamin K-2 and tons of free radical-scavenging ascorbic acid (vitamin C). They provide nearly 300% of your recommended daily vitamin C intake! That's better than the popular orange, considered for decades to be the best source of this essential vitamin.

In addition, red bell peppers contain skin-renewing vitamin A, sight-boosting lutein, lycopene, and beta-carotene. A medium-sized red bell pepper also provides substantial vitamin B6, which helps your body make critical neurotransmitters and lowers breast cancer risk factors.

When buying red bell peppers, be sure to buy organic as these contain higher levels of vitamin C and lutein than those grown conventionally.

Cauliflower the Globe of Hope

Although cauliflower isn't as famous as its cousin kale, it's a proud member of the mustard family. Vegetables such as cauliflower, watercress, cabbage, bok choy, broccoli, kale, horseradish, turnip, rutabaga, arugula, and Brussel sprouts are cruciferous. Studies confirm these vegetables are high in glucosinolates (chemical compounds with anti-cancer properties) and can definitely lower risk of bladder, breast, colon, prostate, and ovarian cancers.

Cruciferous vegetables, so called because of their four petal flowers that resemble crosses, are proven to induce **apoptosis** (cell death or cell suicide) in cancerous cells while leaving normal healthy cells untouched.

A study led by Professor Ah-Ng Tony Kong at Rutgers University revealed that cauliflower is also abundant in sulforaphane (SFN). SFN has been shown to inhibit the occurrence of hereditary cancers often arising from your genetic background.

"Our research has substantiated the connection between diet and cancer prevention, and it is now clear that the expression of cancer-related genes can be influenced by chemo preventative compounds in the things we eat," said Kong, a professor of pharmaceutics in the Ernest Mario School of Pharmacy at Rutgers, The State University of New Jersey.

The study corroborated the research that SFN found in cauliflower and other cruciferous vegetables has chemo preventative activity.

Professor Kong said, "We feel SFN should be evaluated clinically for its chemo preventative potential in patients with related colon cancers."

A Little about Fish

Since the curry recipe is rich and complex in flavor, I've created a simple buttery broiled fish recipe that will deliciously compliment your anti-cancer veggie side.

Remember...always choose sustainable fish sources:

- Cod – wild caught Pacific
- Haddock – line caught, Marine Stewardship Council (MSC) certified sustainable seafood, certified haddock from Scotland, Norway, or other countries
- Pollock – MSC certified from Alaska or other countries
- Wild shrimp or prawns – (not a fish, but a delicious option) MSC certified from Canada, other countries, or wild organic (never buy farmed shrimp)
- Sea bass – line caught and wild organic
- Diver scallops – look for dived scallops (also not a fish, but another delicious option)
- Pacific wild halibut – MSC certified or organic gilthead Bream

Chermoula Broiled Whitefish or Seafood Recipe

Serves 4 / Prep Time: 30 minutes / Cook Time: 60 minutes

Ingredients

- 2 cloves garlic
- 1 cups coriander leaf (loosely packed fresh and tender stems)
- 1 ½ cups Italian parsley leaves (loosely packed fresh and tender stems)
- 1 lemon (divided)
- 6 tablespoons plain geek yogurt
- 1 tablespoon olive oil
- 1 teaspoon ground cumin
- Dash ground cayenne pepper (to taste)
- Dash sea salt (to taste)
- Olive oil or coconut oil
- 20 ounces whitefish fillets (or other filleted seafood you prefer)
- ½ teaspoon fresh ground black pepper

Method

1. Move oven rack 4 inches from heat source and preheat broiler.

2. Prepare chermoula. In food processor, combine garlic, cilantro, parsley and lemon zest and process to finely chop. Add yogurt, lemon juice, oil, paprika, cumin, and cayenne and process to incorporate. Add salt (to taste) and set aside.

3. Use shallow baking dish or large foil-lined baking sheet. Rub bottom with oil. Salt and pepper fish. Spread about a quarter of chermoula on both sides of fish. Arrange fish in baking dish or on sheet in a single layer and set aside at room temperature for 15 minutes.

4. Broil fish until just cooked through, 5 to 7 minutes. Transfer to serving plates and drizzle with any cooking juices. Serve remaining chermoula on the side.

Creamy Anti-Cancer Veggie Curry Recipe

Serves 4 / Prep Time: 30 minutes / Cook Time: 60 minutes

Ingredients

- 2 tablespoons olive oil
- 1 large onion, chopped
- Large piece ginger, grated
- 3 garlic cloves, finely chopped
- ½ teaspoon turmeric
- 1 teaspoon ground cumin
- 1 teaspoon curry powder, or to taste
- 1 can chopped tomatoes (BPA-free)
- ½ teaspoon sugar in the raw
- 2 red bell peppers
- 1 fresh cauliflower, cut into florets
- 2 turnips cut into chunks
- 1 small green chili, halved lengthways
- Squeeze of lemon juice
- Handful coriander, roughly chopped, to serve
- Naan bread and Greek yogurt, to serve (optional)

Method

1. Heat oil in a saucepan. Cook onion for 10 minutes until soft. Add ginger, garlic, turmeric, cumin and curry powder. Cook 1 minute more. Stir in tomatoes and sugar.

2. Add turnips and split chili, seasoning to taste. Cover and gently cook (low or medium low) for 20 minutes.

3. Add cauliflower and peppers. Cook an additional 15 minutes. (Check that cauliflower is tender when pierced with a fork, but take care not to overcook it.) Stir occasionally, until the vegetables are tender – add a few drops of water if you need to, but it is meant to be a dry curry.

4. When vegetables are cooked, remove chili from heat. If you like, stir in a squeeze of lemon juice and scatter with coriander. Serve with your choice of Indian bread and a dollop of yogurt.

Day 3
NOURISH

LIVE LONGER WITH A SURPRISING TIP & PREVENT CANCER WITH THE MUSTARD EFFECT FOUND IN FIVE EVERY DAY SUPERFOODS

Welcome to your third day of Vivid Living. Today, we're going to discuss one of my favorite topics...**SUPERFOODS**!

In addition, I'm going to share how you can live longer with this one surprising tip and prevent cancer with the mustard effect found in five every day superfoods.

Today's lesson (I have to admit) will take more than 10 minutes.

That's because you're cooking one of the fabulous, healthy dinner recipes I gave you tonight! You don't need me to tell you when to make dinner... or do you? *Just kidding...*

Let's get going and plunge into day three!

Superfoods. Just the name alone conjures healing thoughts for me. There's a reason superfoods are named just that. The true state of your health is dictated by your daily diet. Cancer is a good example of the power of food. A nutrient-dense healthy diet can help prevent cancer, since nearly 60% of cancer cases are diet-related. The chart on the next page shows the top everyday superfoods by nutrient density...*watercress scored 100!*

Your body uses food to survive and even the simple process of digestion creates stress on your body.

Why not **love and cherish the only body you have** by understanding how the foods you eat affect your health and how long you live?

How to Live Longer by Limiting When You Eat

A little-known factor that can help you live longer is eating within a specific timeframe of 8-12 hours. This is known as **intermittent fasting** (IF). Before you run away screaming, don't worry.

I'm not telling you to *fast*.

Here's how it works: You give your body *at least* 12 hours when it's not required to process food. For instance, if you wake up at 6am and eat breakfast at 7am, then you stop eating completely for the day by 7pm. That gives your body 12 full hours of rest.

Fascinating results were observed during a study conducted at the National Institute on Aging. Researchers discovered that a calorie-restricted diet in Rhesus monkeys studied for 20 years notably decreased and/or delayed the onset of age-related diseases and increased longevity by a factor of three.

In a 2002 study named Comprehensive Assessment of Long-Term Effects of Reducing Intake of Energy (CALERIE), human participants took part in moderate calorie restriction and after one year lowered their fasting glucose, total cholesterol, core body temperature, body weight, and fat.

Here's where it gets interesting! At the cellular level, calorie restriction had an anti-aging effect. The participants reduced their DNA damage and had better functioning mitochondria (the little power factories for your cells).

Intermittent fasting provides a similar benefit to caloric restriction. Your metabolism runs more efficiently, utilizing your consumed food energy before switching to burning fat.

Top Everyday Superfood Fruits and Vegetables by Nutrient Density

Item	Nutrient Density Score
Watercress	100.00
Chinese cabbage	91.99
Chard	89.27
Beet green	87.08
Spinach	86.43
Chicory	73.36
Leaf lettuce	70.73
Parsley	65.59
Romaine lettuce	63.48
Collard green	62.49
Turnip green	62.12
Mustard green	61.39
Endive	60.44
Chive	54.80
Kale	49.07
Dandelion green	46.34
Red pepper	41.26
Arugula	37.65
Broccoli	34.89
Pumpkin	33.82

Item	Nutrient Density Score
Brussels sprout	32.23
Scallion	27.35
Kohlrabi	25.92
Cauliflower	25.13
Cabbage	24.51
Carrot	22.60
Tomato	20.37
Lemon	18.72
Iceberg lettuce	18.28
Strawberry	17.59
Radish	16.91
Winter squash (all varieties)	13.89
Orange	12.91
Lime	12.23
Grapefruit (pink and red)	11.64
Rutabaga	11.58
Turnip	11.43
Blackberry	11.39
Leek	10.69
Sweet potato	10.51
Grapefruit (white)	10.47

Unfortunately, calorie restriction or intermittent fasting won't fortify your body against disease, or we could just eat fewer milkshakes and French fries. You should be limiting those kinds of foods anyway. If you're still consuming a high-refined carbohydrate, low-nutrient diet, this places you in harm's way. Poor eating habits dramatically increases your risk of cancer, Alzheimer's disease, dementia, heart disease, obesity, and type II diabetes.

Refined, calorie-dense deadly foods are everywhere! You have to be the one who takes back the control of your health by actively working to increase your lifespan instead of shortening it.

By replacing an over-processed, high-sugar, carbohydrate-heavy diet with nutrient-packed superfoods in the form of vegetables and proteins, you can extend your lifespan and prevent chronic disease.

Regular fruits and vegetables are good for you (absolutely). However, considering the nutrient content of our soil in the United States has been depleted by nearly 50% from what it was in 1950, the nutritional content you find in today's tomato pales in comparison to the tomato your grandmother used in her meals.

You have to give yourself a winning hand so that the foods you choose work harder to keep you healthy. Superfoods are **50 to 100 times more powerful** than regular fruits and vegetables.

Researcher Jennifer Di Noia, PhD at William Paterson University in New Jersey, helped us all by creating a comprehensive list of 41 superfood fruits and vegetables (found on the previous pages).

These everyday superfoods are scored by their content of fiber, potassium, protein, calcium, folate, vitamin B12, vitamin A, vitamin D, and other essential nutrients.

Basically, this is your "stacked deck" when it comes to nutrition.

By generously sprinkling these superfoods into your daily eating plan, your body will receive the nutrition it needs without all the deceptive "low fat," "sugar-free," and "whole grain" labels that are slapped on food to make you believe it's good for you.

Prevent Cancer with the Mustard Effect Found in Five Everyday Superfoods

You know vegetables can *prevent* cancer but is possible they can *cure* it?

Let's talk about the mustard effect found in cruciferous vegetables (commonly called the mustard family – broccoli, cauliflower, cabbage, watercress, kale, Swiss chard, spinach, Brussel sprouts, bok choy, turnips, rutabaga, arugula, and radishes all belong to the club).

These veggies don't like cancer cells – especially prostate, breast, uterine, and ovarian cancers – and work hard to banish the nasty little destroyers.

Does that sound too good to be true?

There are over 120 peer-reviewed scientific studies on indol-3-carbinol (I3C) – the outstanding phytochemical found these cancer-fighting veggies.

Studies from Wayne State University School of Medicine, in Detroit, Michigan found that I3C functions as an **inhibitor and chemotherapeutic agent** for prostate cancer.

Cancers such as breast, uterine, and ovarian cancers feed on estrogen. Instead of attacking cancer cells, I3C **reverses their ability to convert estrogen** from "bad" to "good."

• *Bad estrogen* – feeds cancer in breast and reproductive tissues.

• *Good estrogen* – stops this out of control cell growth.

Since the type of estrogen your body makes creates a difference, I3C is critical in inhibiting and down-regulating the responses of estrogen-responsive genes.

The antitumor activities of I3C regulate estrogen, metabolism, and the estrogen receptor. These play an important role in the spread of breast cancer cells and tumor development, as discovered by the Department of Radiation and Oncology at Long Island Jewish Medical Center in New Hyde Park, New York.

You can easily incorporate these five everyday cancer-fighting superfoods in your weeknight dinners.

I've created delicious (easy to follow) recipes that serve four people. There's also a separate downloadable recipe sheet and grocery list.

DAY THREE DINNER

QUINOA, GRAPEFRUIT, BEET GREENS & FETA SALAD

Strengthen Your Bones with Beneficial Beet Greens

Ancient Romans loved beet greens but threw away the roots! It wasn't discovered until much later that you could actually eat the roots.

Today, it's the opposite. Most of us love the ruby red sweetness of beet roots. Get ready to love the beet green!

These delicate greens provide a powerful amount of magnesium, potassium, copper, manganese, and 220% of your recommended daily vitamin A.

The goodness of beet greens doesn't stop there...

Beet greens help prevent osteoporosis and work together with calcium to **improve bone density** and strength.

Since beet greens are higher in iron than spinach, they can help to **relieve fatigue**, oxygenate the blood, and aid in necessary blood clotting.

Did you know...beet greens contain tryptophan? I bet you thought it was only found in turkey! Tryptophan helps produce the "feel good" chemical serotonin, which **regulates mood** and sleep cycles.

Beet greens are also great for **detoxifying the liver** of heavy metals, excess calcium, pesticides, and can help strengthen the vascular system.

Beet greens wilt easily, so be sure to use them within 2-3 days of purchase.

Quinoa, Grapefruit, Beet Greens & Feta Salad

Serves 4 / Prep Time: 50 minutes / Cook Time: 35 minutes

Ingredients

- ½ cup raw quinoa (any variety) (if you don't eat quinoa, you can swap with 3 cups of diced oven-roasted potatoes for a delicious substitute.)
- ¾ cup water
- 1 bunch beetroots (4 medium, roasted)
- 1 pound beet greens (from your bunch)
- Salt & pepper (to taste)
- 2 tablespoons extra-virgin olive oil
- 3 garlic cloves (minced)
- 1 tablespoon oregano
- 4 ounces feta cheese
- 1 pink (or any variety) grapefruit, peeled and sliced (save some juice)

Method

1. Scrub, dice, and roast beets (350 degrees for 45 mins). Peeling is optional (but unnecessary). Once cooled, set aside.

2. Rinse quinoa thoroughly with cold water. Use a sieve. (Note: always rinse quinoa before cooking or it has a slightly grassy taste.)

3. Place quinoa and water in a medium pot. Cover and bring to a boil. Once boiling, turn down to simmer for 11 minutes. Stir and let sit covered an additional 5 minutes.

4. Fluff with a fork and place in large glass or ceramic bowl.

5. Blanch greens in a large pot of generously salted water or steam them above an inch of boiling water until wilted, one to two minutes. Refresh with cold water, squeeze dry and chop.

6. Heat olive oil over medium heat in a large, heavy skillet. Add garlic. Cook, stirring, until fragrant, 30 seconds to a minute. Add oregano, beet greens, and salt and pepper to taste. Stir over medium heat for 30 seconds to a minute until the greens are nicely infused.

7. Add beets and quinoa. Toss together until the ingredients are well combined and the quinoa is heated through and colored with beet juice. Taste and adjust salt and pepper.

8. Transfer to a wide serving bowl or platter, let cool for 10 minutes. Add feta cheese and sliced grapefruit.

9. Mix 2 tablespoons of extra virgin olive oil and 1 tablespoon of fresh grapefruit juice, drizzle over salad, toss lightly, and season to taste with salt and pepper.

Day 4
REBUILD

CREATIVE VISUALIZATION

HOW YOUR THOUGHTS AFFECT YOUR BEHAVIORS, LIFE, AND OUTCOMES

In our fast-paced world, would you believe that the secret to getting what you desire in life is to actually *slow down* and *visualize* it?

Today I'm going to discuss how you can increase your happiness and create positive change in your mental and emotional well-being.

It's so easily overlooked and it has EVERYTHING to do with your thoughts...

Your thoughts create your feelings, your feelings influence your actions, and your actions provide end results. If your life isn't where you want it to be, changing your thoughts is the first step to getting what you truly want.

Visualization is a cognitive technique that allows you to access your imagination in order to realize all your life's desires.

There are many different visualization techniques, but the most effective ones allow you to mentally *rehearse* or *imagine* an action in order to bring your entire mind and body to a state of relaxation.

Through this practice, you can picture your ideal life. Once you accomplish the vision, you can start taking the necessary steps to fulfill your dreams.

Your beliefs create your reality. Often, what you *believe* to be true of the world around you is crucial...because you *influence* it.

To get the most out of this unit, don't worry about the differing viewpoints on visualization. Instead, focus on the scientifically proven evidence confirming that what you visualize with your mind tends to shape your personal reality.

This is a powerful message. It means your mind has a degree of control over both your own body as well as the literal path of your own life.

Let's look at a powerful visualization experiment conducted by Soviet sports scientists as well as the findings studied by Dr. Charles Garfield, a former NASA researcher.

Back in the 1980's, the study examined the effect of mental training, including visualization, on athletes at the Lake Placid Olympics.

The athletes were divided into four groups:

- Group one did 100% physical training

- Group two did 75% physical training and 25% mental technique

- Group three did equal parts physical and mental training

- Group four did 25% physical training and 75% mental technique

Which group of athletes do you think did the best? *Go on guess...I'll wait.*

Are you ready for the answer? It was group four! *Shocking, I know!* In fact, all the groups that utilized mental training along with physical training out-performed group one, which only used physical training. Group three did better than group two and group two better than group one.

Garfield explained, "During mental rehearsal, athletes create mental images of the exact movements they want to emulate in their sport. Use of this skill substantially increases the effectiveness of goal-setting, which up until then had been little more than a dull listing procedure."

If mental exercises and visualization could have such a profound impact on Olympic athletes, improving their performance so effectively, what kind of impact could it have on you?

That's the power of creative visualization.

Through visualization, you can drastically change your mindset, become a happier, well-adjusted person, and ultimately get what you want out of life.

Don't worry about the *road*, just trust in *the process* that your end goal will be realized.

There's another important key to making creative visualization work. In order to get what you want, you have to know *exactly* what you want.

You must be specific in your visualizations...to ensure you get precisely what you visualize.

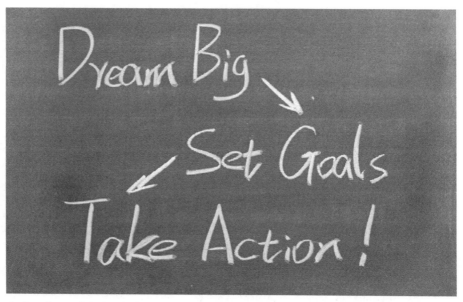

It begins with belief, followed by visualizations, and carried through to actions.

Too often, our minds work for us in negative ways. We create negative outcomes because we visualize a situation in a negative way. That's what happens when you're guided by fear, anxiety, or lack of confidence.

It's time to tap into your true potential! Use the power of visualization to create the positive outcomes you truly want.

This practice shouldn't be confused with "faith" or "positive thinking."

Creative visualization creates "coincidences" that move you toward your goals. Don't worry about the *how* – the steps to get you there. That part is important but it isn't your motivation.

Focus only on *what* you want.

By changing your overall mindset about yourself, your life, and the world around you through creative visualization, you can experience the following benefits:

Become the Person You Have Always Wanted to Be

I'm sure you have an "ideal" of the person you want to become. With visualization, you can become the best version of you and achieve the success you desire in life.

Envision how you would interact with others, how you would respond to challenges, how you would create your successes – then use those mental scenes you've created and imitate them as your new model of behavior.

Permanently Boost Self-Confidence

Without self-confidence, you won't believe you are capable of achieving your dreams. The *inner belief* that you are *worthy* of your dreams, your happiness, and your desires – that is the core of confidence.

Through visualization, you can boost your self-confidence and keep moving towards your goals.

Achieve Your Dream Life

You have goals – both large and small – that you want to achieve in life. Through this practice, you can subconsciously reprogram your mental models so that you start to create the right mindset that enables you to work towards your dreams.

Visualization allows you to stop subconsciously sabotaging yourself so you can focus on the aspects of your life and future that truly matter.

Become a Person Others Can Count On

Being a person that your family and friends can count on is a wonderful feeling. However, being that person for *yourself* is priceless.

When you do what you say, living up to promises you make yourself, your integrity and actions resonate to your family and friends. You become a pillar of strength for yourself and for them.

Keys to Practice Creative Visualization...

Through creative visualization techniques, you can teach your brain to achieve the success that you desire in all of the aspects of your life. It's time to abolish a lifetime of negative self-talk, lack of confidence in your abilities, and hesitation about seizing what you want.

1. **Remove subconscious negative sabotage.** Maybe you've received input (as most of us have) since early childhood such as you're not "lucky enough" to have money, that you "aren't the type" to do that, or "life is hard" so dreams aren't valid.

   These messages become hardwired into our thinking. Over time, we end up *believing* statements like these and they ultimately *become* our reality.

   In order to change your reality, you need to be aware of the subconscious aspects of your existing reality. These subconscious beliefs – about yourself and the world around you – influence *how others perceive you* and *how you perceive everything* in your life.

2. **You can create a new reality by defining exactly what you want it to be.** You wouldn't go on a trip and buy three different airline tickets to three different destinations, would you? No, when it comes to travel, you know exactly where you are going, how you will get there, where you will stay, and for how long.

   In order to get what you want in other parts of your life, this same *clarity* and *sense of purpose* is crucial. It will take time, it will take your undivided attention, but don't quit. Stay focused and determined that you will do it.

3. **Don't feel guilty about what you want.** There's nothing more damaging than guilt. You are powerful, fierce, and beautiful...guilt has no place in your new reality.

   Don't simply visualize doing well in a job interview. Instead, visualize the home you'll buy for your family with the better job you're determined to win. Visualize the experience you'll get from that new job, the security it will provide, and the happiness it will give you and your family.

See it clearly, know this is the first step to move you closer to your goals, and then *take the steps* to achieve what you want. Visualization without action doesn't work!

4. **Dream big!** Don't be afraid to think outside the box.

    Remember, at this stage, you're not supposed to worry about the *how*. Visualize what you want and take actions to get yourself to your desired goals. Expect that the things you want to happen – *will* happen.

5. **Go into every situation expecting to win.** You will be shocked at how effective this simple mindset will be. When you *believe in your personal ability to win* at anything, more often than not, it turns into a self-fulfilling prophecy.

    Stop worrying. Trust in the process and know that your desires are rightfully yours. Feel that what you desire is already yours. It is already yours.

6. **Express gratitude for what you have.** The importance of gratitude cannot be stressed more strongly. When you are truly grateful for what you have – no matter how "small" you feel it is – you understand that you could have "less."

    When you embrace this concept, you also recognize that having "more" is within your power. Gratitude for what you already have as well as what you will attain is critical.

Are you ready to start visualizing?

I'm going to give you two basic creative visualization exercises. Your homework for today is to pick one to try. People respond better to different types of visualization techniques. If one isn't right for you, use the other.

Treasure Map Visualization

This visualization technique utilizes both your physical and mental capacities.

To begin, think of something that you want to occur in your life – such as getting a better job, moving to another place, or finding your romantic partner.

Write out, draw, choose an object, or print a picture – a physical representation of your desire – and meditate on the picture, words, or object for at least three minutes every day.

Receptive Visualization

This technique involves only using your mental facilities.

To begin, sit or lie down in a quiet area. Use your imagination to visualize a scene you want to occur in your future. It's similar to creating a mental short film. See yourself in the scene, doing what you want most, and fix it firmly in your mind.

Over time, you'll add more detail or take some aspects away, until you have the ideal meditation image. Meditate on these images daily to achieve your dreams.

Creative visualization is a scientifically based practice that engages the power of your mind to help you become the person that you desire.

Through *visualization* and *actions*, you can achieve your personal goals. The first step to attaining true fulfillment and happiness is *believing* and *seeing* that outcome in your own mind.

Again, your homework today is to do just ONE of the visualization exercises. Until tomorrow, continue to live vividly!

DAY FOUR DINNER

EASY STIR-FRIED CHINESE CABBAGE WITH BACON OR COOL CABBAGE MANGO SLAW WITH WILD SHRIMP

Safeguard Your Stomach & Prevent Cancer with Chinese Cabbage

Sulfur-containing glucosinolates that give plants like cabbage and horse-radish their bite are broken down in the small intestine and colon within 2 to 3 hours of eating. Eating cabbage with gusto can help protect against cancers of the lung and alimentary tract that extends from your mouth to anus. This was studied by the Institute of Food Research in Norwich, England.

The *Encyclopedia of Healing Foods* by Michael Murray, N.D. and Joseph Pizzorno, N.D., found that the glucosinolates in cabbage increase the body's antioxidant defense mechanisms, improve its detoxification ability, and assist in eliminating harmful chemicals and hormones.

Indole-3-carbinole (I3C) increases the rate at which estrogen (found in numerous plastics and personal care products), steroid hormones, carcinogens, toxins, and drugs break down through the liver's detoxification process by nearly 50%. I3C even helps to inhibit the development of stomach, colon, prostate, and breast cancers while also healing peptic ulcers.

Easy Stir-Fried Chinese Cabbage with Bacon

Serves 4 / Prep Time: 30 minutes / Cook Time: 10 minutes

Ingredients

- 1 pound green cabbage, halved, cored, and torn into bite-size pieces (or finely chopped)

- 2 tablespoons Chinkiang vinegar (sold in Asian Supermarkets; if not available, use 1 tablespoon of red wine vinegar and 1 tablespoon of apple cider vinegar)
- 1 teaspoon soy sauce or coconut aminos
- 4 strips thick-cut bacon, cut into ¼ inch pieces
- 2 to 3 fresh cayenne chili peppers or other fresh red chili, thinly sliced on the bias with seeds
- 3 medium cloves garlic, thinly sliced lengthwise
- 2 scallions cut into 1-inch pieces on the bias
- ½ of a red onion diced
- 1 pound of cremini mushrooms
- 1 pound of shiitake mushrooms

Method

1. Fill a wok or a large pot with water and bring to boil. Add cabbage and cook until crisp-tender, about 1 minute. Drain in a colander and rinse with cold running water; press cabbage to expel any excess water.

2. In a small bowl, combine Chinkiang vinegar and soy sauce. Mix and set aside.

3. In a wok, cook bacon over high heat until golden brown, about 3-5 minutes. Using a slotted spoon or spider, transfer bacon to paper towel-lined plate. Pour off all but 1 tablespoon of rendered bacon fat from wok. Reserve 1 extra tablespoon.

4. Using the bacon fat to sauté diced onions and mushrooms, about 2 minutes. Remove from wok.

5. Heat wok over high heat with reserved bacon fat until lightly smoking. Add chilies, garlic, and scallions. Stir-fry until garlic is golden, about 30 seconds. Toss in cabbage and stir-fry until warmed through.

6. Add vinegar mixture, bacon, onions, and mushrooms. Continue to stir-fry until cabbage is tender, about 2 minutes. Transfer to a serving plate and serve immediately.

Cool Cabbage Mango Slaw
with Wild Shrimp

Serves 4 / Prep Time: 30 minutes / Cook Time: 10 minutes

Ingredients

- 2 cups shredded cabbage
- ½ cup shredded carrots
- ½ cup julienned dried figs
- 1 mango, almost fully ripe
- 2 medium scallions, chopped
- 3 tablespoons rice vinegar
- ½ lime, juiced
- 1 tablespoon soy sauce (use tamari for gluten-free or coconut amino)
- 1 tablespoon sesame oil
- 1 teaspoon black and white sesame seeds
- 1 ½ pounds of peeled wild shrimp

Method

1. Boil shrimp for 5 minutes until pink. Drain and rinse with cool water. Peel shrimp (if not already peeled). Once shrimp are cooled, refrigerate until ready to serve.

2. Julienne mango (cut into strips). Combine with cabbage, carrots, scallions, and fig. Toss well in a large bowl.

3. Prepare dressing by combining rice vinegar, soy sauce, and lime juice; slowly include the oil. Whisk thoroughly.

4. Pour dressing immediately over cabbage mixture and toss well to coat. Let it sit for 20 minutes to allow the slaw to marinate.

5. Add shrimp and sesame seeds, mix well, and serve!

Day 5
DETOXIFY

DETOXIFY YOUR BODY & BOOST YOUR IMMUNITY

So far, we've covered hydration to refresh you, poses to empower you, food to nourish you, and visualization to keep you focused on your dreams.

Other than cooking, you're still only investing a few minutes every day towards the life of your dreams...the *vivid life* that you deserve.

Today, we're going to talk about protecting your most valuable asset. It's your first line of defense against sickness and disease. It's also your body's largest organ: **your skin**.

The skin that covers you is sometimes referred to as the "third kidney." It earned this reputation because it's responsible for 10-15% of waste elimination **and** total body detoxification.

Your skin, as your internal organs, can become congested or clogged as toxins build up from poor nutrition, lack of sleep, prolonged stress, pollution, and heavy metals.

Toxic buildup can manifest in the following symptoms:
- Unexplained fatigue
- Low-grade inflammation
- Mental fog
- Bloating
- Allergies
- Puffy skin or eyes

Not only is this toxic build-up dangerous to your health, it can create an excess of melanin in the skin creating hyperpigmentation and blotchy skin tone.

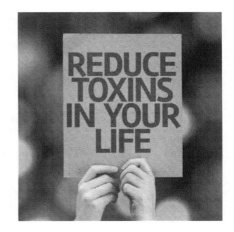

Your skin is the number one protective barrier that prevents toxins from entering your body. When it's compromised, you need to repair it with a simple detox lifestyle practice.

Instead of waking up and grabbing your usual cup of coffee, there's an alternative routine that's just as rejuvenating that can improve your life in ways you might not have considered.

Dry skin brushing is a swift and powerful way to enhance the detoxification process. It's easy, pleasant, and yields tremendous benefits – such as brushing away days of accumulated stress, tension, and toxins!

Every minute, we lose over 30,000 dead skin cells. Those are being constantly replaced by healthy new cells. As the new skin gets closer to the surface, many of the toxins inside you are pushed upwards as well, toward the outside of your body.

It is a *brilliant* yet *simple* method of detoxification that happens naturally.

Not only does dry brushing improve the appearance of your skin by eliminating dead skin cells, it helps new skin to regenerate and increases blood circulation that aids in eliminating toxins.

An added bonus is that the massaging effect of the bristles reduces the appearance of cellulite!

Dry brushing stimulates internal circulation, boosts lymphatic drainage, and firms the skin by encouraging collagen growth. The increase in efficient blood circulation improves brain function and raises energy levels.

The Importance of the Lymph System

Your lymphatic system is composed of lymph vessels that are larger than your blood vessels. It is your body's waste removal and immune system. It regulates your fat, protein, water, and waste disposal.

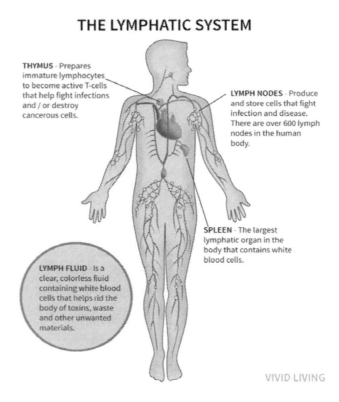

THE LYMPHATIC SYSTEM

THYMUS - Prepares immature lymphocytes to become active T-cells that help fight infections and / or destroy cancerous cells.

LYMPH NODES - Produce and store cells that fight infection and disease. There are over 600 lymph nodes in the human body.

SPLEEN - The largest lymphatic organ in the body that contains white blood cells.

LYMPH FLUID - Is a clear, colorless fluid containing white blood cells that helps rid the body of toxins, waste and other unwanted materials.

VIVID LIVING

It's such a crucial part of your overall health and it's time to stop ignoring it! Give it the love and attention it deserves.

You've probably seen your lymph fluid when you've had a cut. It's the pale yellow fluid that seeps from a wound after bleeding. You've also probably felt a swollen lymph node (beneath your jaw, under your arms, or in your groin) if you've suffered from an infection.

Functions of the Lymph System:

- Removes large fat and protein particles from the small intestine through lymph vessels called the 'lacteals.'

- Lymph contains white blood cells called lymphocytes, which are regulated by lymph nodes to fight disease, sickness, and infections.

- Lymph vessels carry waste material up the thoracic duct. It goes back into the blood vessels by linking up with the main vein of the heart. Then the waste is transported by blood and excreted out through the lungs, skin, kidneys, and bowels.

- Controls water flow in and out of cells, since we are 75% water, our lymphatic system removes up to 2.5 liters of fluid per day from our cells. Lymph nodes act as filters and cleansing service stations for your body's waste.

- The lymph system is vital to a healthy and balanced immune system response. It relies on skeletal muscle contractions to help pump it and assist lymph flow.

To keep your lymph system functioning efficiently, dry skin brushing is the ultimate detoxing technique that is easy to do in the privacy of your own home. There are no side effects, no "potions" to apply or drink, and it is safe for use at any age.

How to Dry Brush Detox

You will need a natural stiff-bristled bath or shower brush with a long handle. You can find these at a natural health food store or a home goods store. If your skin is very sensitive, go with a slightly softer brush. The long handle will help you easily reach all your body parts.

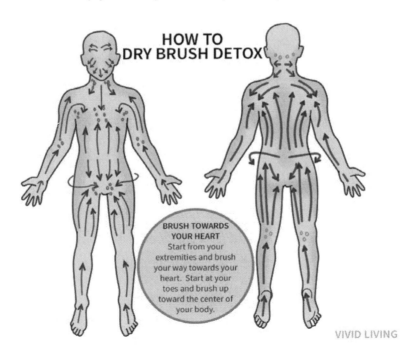

Stand in the bathtub or on a towel. The best time to dry brush is just before a shower or bath. Always start on dry skin.

Start from your extremities and brush your way *towards* your heart. Start at your toes and brush up toward the center of your body. When dry brushing your stomach, brush in a clockwise motion since that mimics your natural digestive flow.

It may tingle at first or even tickle but don't stop! You're going to feel rejuvenated and energized when you're done! Don't use the dry-brushing technique on your face or on skin that is broken, cut, burned, or injured.

Enjoy your new glow and know that you're also assisting your lymphatic system to prevent pain, inflammation, circulatory, and immune system disorders.

Bonus Tip

Follow a dry brushing session with a simple hydrotherapy technique. Hydrotherapy helps increase circulation and reduces inflammation. It temporarily expands and then constricts the blood vessels. This relaxes the muscles and reduces pain, muscle spasms, and fatigue.

Take a hot shower (as hot as you can stand) for five minutes. Stand completely under the showerhead and allow the water to flow down your back. Follow with cold water for 30 seconds. Return to hot water for one minute, cold water for 30 seconds, repeating three times in total. After you dry off, climb into your bed for 30 minutes.

Your homework today is to dry brush your skin before your bath or shower. You're going to be amazed at how it makes you feel! You'll feel like you've spent the day at the spa!

Until tomorrow...live your life vividly!

WHY YOU NEED TO TRY A LYMPHATIC CLEANSE

By now, you know your beautiful lymph system is *critical* to your health. If you haven't considered a lymphatic cleanse, let me show you why it should be part of your healthy lifestyle!

The care and keeping of your lymphatic system directly affects the condition of your immune system, digestion, central nervous system, and how your body handles toxins found in your food, water, and air.

It is an underlying (and often misdiagnosed) cause of many health crisis – including cancer. If the vessels become blocked or stop working - lymph fluid builds up in your body. This can happen when your body is overwhelmed with toxins and the lymph system is unable to keep up.

Bacteria and other waste build up because the lymph system isn't flushing them out. These waste products build up in the nodes.

Your breathing and body movement is the power source behind your lymphatic system and you will die within mere hours if it stops functioning. It works hand-in-hand with your gut and both determine your overall wellness.

You should always let your regular doctor know before you do any type of cleanse – especially if you're under medical care for a chronic condition.

Avoid manufactured cleanses because they are usually filled with chemicals and other ingredients that *force* a reaction from your body. Natural, common-sense methods are safer (and more effective).

The cleanse we suggest takes three days.

As you'll see, this is based on safe, natural ingredients that boost all the cells in your body with abundant nutrients.

During the cleanse, avoid alcohol, tobacco, excess sugar, too much coffee, and "white" foods such as pasta, rice, wheat, or sugar. Drink *at least* 64 ounces of water daily.

3-Day Natural Lymphatic Cleanse Recipe

You will need...

- Organic vegetables (mostly green) that include zucchini, celery, greens, cabbage, peppers, kale, spinach, carrots, beets, onions, and garlic cloves
- Two gallons of distilled water
- Large stockpot with lid
- Large strainer and pot
- Glass containers – enough to hold two gallons of broth

Directions...

- Wash veggies thoroughly but do not peel (with exception to garlic).
- In a large pot, combine all vegetables with two gallons of distilled water.
- Bring to a boil then turn to low heat.
- Cover the pot and simmer for two hours.
- Remove from heat and allow to cool completely.
- Strain the vegetables from the liquid (these will be reused later so save and refrigerate), leaving only the liquid behind.
- Store the vegetable broth in glass jars in your refrigerator.

Day One – Lymphatic Cleanse

- Drink three glasses (8 ounces each) of broth before lunch.
- Drink three glasses (8 ounces each) of broth before dinner.

Day Two – Lymphatic Cleanse

- Drink three glasses (8 ounces each) of broth before breakfast.
- Drink three glasses (8 ounces each) of broth before lunch.
- Drink three glasses (8 ounces each) of broth before dinner.

Day Three – Lymphatic Cleanse

- Drink three glasses (8 ounces each) of broth before breakfast.
- Drink three glasses (8 ounces each) of broth before lunch.

Include the boiled vegetables you removed from the broth during preparation in your evening meal. These can be prepared in whatever way you wish.

Add enough distilled water to your original broth to ensure you have enough for the day.

Detoxifying and cleansing your body naturally has been done for thousands of years and it is going to change your life – how you feel today and how your body responds for decades to come. A lymphatic cleanse is a major step in preventative care and quality of life.

As with every true step toward good health, a strong lymphatic system requires daily healthy lifestyle choices that you probably already know (but are hesitant to implement).

3 Steps to a Healthier Lymph System Every Day

1. **Eat cleanly.** When you fill your body with processed foods, sodas, hydrogenated oils, or refined flours and sugars, you increase the amount of toxins that the lymph system has to flush. If it is sold in a box or found on the frozen meals aisle in your market, chances are, it isn't good for you.

   Choosing organic whole foods that include lots of fruits and vegetables, healthy fats, water, and lean meats will give your body clean fuel to burn with less toxic burden.

2. **Take food sensitivity seriously.** Eliminate foods or other items that don't "sit well" with your stomach. Increase your intake of probiotic foods to strengthen healthy gut flora.

   A strong digestive system is crucial to total body wellness as well as neurological function, heart health, and immunity.

3. **Get moving.** Your lymph system only works when you do. The lymph vessels pump *against gravity* and are powered by the muscle contractions in your body.

Not getting any sort of consistent exercise will result in sluggish lymphatic function. If possible, get exercise, fresh air, and sunshine (for incredible vitamin D) at the same time!

Don't stop there!

Doing this 2-4 times per year is going to change how you feel. It literally allows your lymphatic system to "reset" and clear out the excess waste from your body.

After the cleanse, ease into your usual eating habits slowly. The cleanse broth fills you up (with your water as well) and you probably ate very little solid food for three days.

To keep your lymph system running strong between cleanses, incorporate a glass of distilled (room temperature) water each morning with the juice of half a lemon.

Lymph massages are wonderful but if you don't have the access or means, incorporate a daily dry-brushing detox between lymphatic cleanses.

Stretch, breathe deeply several times each day, and get the sleep you need. Your lymph system – your entire body – will thank you with many more decades of faithful service.

DAY FIVE DINNER

GARLIC ROSEMARY LAMB CHOPS WITH BELUGA LENTILS & CHARD

Why Eat Swiss Chard? Boost Endurance, Lower Blood Pressure, & Control Diabetes with Swiss Chard

Did you know if you're over age 50, your blood pressure naturally increases?

The increase is due to structural changes in the arteries and sometimes due to large artery stiffness. High blood pressure doesn't just select those of us who are a bit older. If you're a man under the age of 45, you're more likely to have high blood pressure. If you're a woman over age 65, then you're at greater risk of having high blood pressure.

1-in-3 adults in the United States have high blood pressure.

Even if you haven't been diagnosed with high blood pressure, **you could still be at risk.** In most cases of high blood pressure, there are no symptoms and there is no known cause.

High blood pressure is a silent killer. It can lead to brain damage, weaken your arteries, damage your liver and kidneys, and tragically even cause heart failure.

Swiss chard or chard is packed with calcium, magnesium, and potassium – these minerals help lower blood pressure by releasing sodium from the body.

According to a study published in the *British Journal of Clinical Pharmacology*, foods high in dietary nitrates like Swiss chard have been shown to have multiple vascular benefits, including reducing blood pressure, preventing platelet clotting, and improving endothelial dysfunction – which usually signals cardiovascular risks.

Swiss chard (also called spinach beet, crab beet, mangold, or silver beet) also lowers the amount of oxygen needed during exercise and has been shown to boost athletic endurance and performance.

It can even help those suffering from cardiovascular, respiratory, or metabolic disease to oxygenate the blood and ease the exertion when it comes to the daily activities of life.

Another powerful compound found in chard is alpha-lipoic acid (ALA), which can lower glucose levels, increase insulin sensitivity, and decrease nerve damage in diabetics. Raw Swiss chard packs more than **300% of your daily requirement for vitamin K** in a one-cup serving!

To get the maximum benefits of cruciferous vegetables and to protect your thyroid, always cook your crucifers. Most cruciferous vegetables are high in oxalic acid, which can bind with minerals in the body and cause them to crystallize. This process can lead to the creation of kidney stones.

They are also goitrogenic, meaning they can inhibit the uptake of iodine by the thyroid gland. An easy way to decrease the goitrogens by about 90% is to boil these beneficial veggies for 3-5 minutes.

Discard the cooking water and enjoy!

Garlic Rosemary Lamb Chops

Serves 4 / Prep Time: 30 minutes / Marinating Time: 1-4 hours / Cook Time: 60 minutes

Ingredients

- 8 lamb chops (2 pounds or 32 ounces)
- Zest of 1 lemon
- 3 tablespoons olive oil
- 1 garlic clove, minced
- 1 tablespoon dried oregano
- 2 tablespoons fresh rosemary leaves, minced
- ¼ teaspoon crushed red pepper flakes
- ¼ teaspoon salt

Method

1. Place the lamb chops into a gallon-sized Ziploc bag. Place on a platter or large plate.

2. Add the remaining ingredients to the bag and close securely. Use your hands to combine the ingredients in the bag and cover the lamb chops. Add more olive oil, if the marinade looks dry.

3. Refrigerate for at least 1 hour and up to 4 hours.

4. Preheat a grill pan or grill over medium heat. (If using a grill pan turn on your stove vent or hood, or open a window)

5. Add 4 lamb chops to the middle of the grill pan and sear for 3 minutes. Flip with tongs and sear the other side for 3 – 4 minutes. Use the tongs to press the fatty side of the lamb and bone of the chop against the hot grill pan – this will sear off any blood and crisp up the fat.

6. Place the chops on a platter or cutting board and allow to rest for at least 15 minutes. Repeat with the remaining lamb chops. (Note: this will cook your lamb to medium – if you want medium rare, decrease the time to 3 minutes on one side and 2 – 3 minutes on the other).

Beluga Lentils & Swiss Chard

Serves 4 / Prep Time: 30 minutes / Marinating Time: 1-4 hours / Cook Time: 60 minutes

Ingredients

-   4 shiitake mushroom caps
-   3 cloves garlic, peeled and minced
-   Salt and freshly ground black pepper
-   1 whole garlic clove
-   1 medium yellow onion, whole
-   1 medium onion, diced
-   1 bay leaf
-   2 ½ cups organic chicken stock
-   ½ pound beluga lentils, picked over and rinsed
-   2 pounds Swiss chard

- 2 tablespoons ghee
- 1 tablespoon of finely chopped sage

Method

1. Press clove into onion and place onion in a medium saucepan with bay leaf, stock, lentils, and a pinch of salt. Bring to a boil over high heat. Reduce heat to medium and simmer, skimming occasionally, until lentils are tender, 30–35 minutes. Discard onion and bay leaf. Set lentils aside.

2. In a large saucepan, add one tablespoon ghee and cooked chard stems, diced onions, and garlic. Stir for one minute, then add leaves, mushroom caps (once the stems are a bit tender), and sage. Adjust seasoning, and cook for 3 minutes. Stir in lentils and remaining ghee.

3. Serve lamb chops and lentils with Swiss chard.

How to cook Swiss Chard

1. Use a large pot (3 quart) with lots of water. Make sure water is at rapid boil before adding Swiss chard.

2. Cut off tough, bottom part of Swiss chard stems.

3. Add the chopped leaves to the boiling water. Do not cover. Cook for 3 minutes; begin timing as soon as you drop the Swiss chard into the boiling water.

4. Place in colander and press out excess water.

5. Toss with rest of ingredients while Chard is still hot.

Day 6
REVITALIZE

ONE SIMPLE SUPERFOOD THAT WILL REVITALIZE YOUR BODY & HOW TO LIMIT EXPOSURE TO FOUR COMMON EVERYDAY TOXINS

How are you feeling? Did you enjoy yesterday's homework?

Dry brushing is a powerful practice that will help you to detoxify naturally. I hope you tried dry brushing as your new 10-minute daily detox practice. If you didn't do it yesterday, take the time before you shower or bath to give yourself a little dry brushing love.

Today, I'm going to share several ways you can help your body detox as well as keep your home sparkling clean without harmful chemicals or toxins.

I call it Revitalize and this unit will help renew every cell in your body with one of the most powerful and perfect superfoods on the planet. You'll also discover how to purify your home with non-toxic cleaners.

Let's get started.

By now, you know that every day you're bombarded with toxins from dangerous household cleaners, personal hygiene products, air fresheners, pesticides, pollution, and processed foods. Some of them are found in things considered "safe" and that makes them especially dangerous.

Common Toxic Offender #1 - Fluoride

Fluoride is found in toothpaste, fluoridated water, and non-organic food. "Conventionally grown iceberg lettuce can contain as much as 180ppm of fluoride – 180 times *higher* than what's recommended in drinking water," says Dr. Joseph Mercola.

Fluoridation caused approximately 10,000 cancer deaths according to epidemiological studies conducted by Dr. Dean Burk, former chief of the Cytochemistry Section for 30 years at the National Cancer Institute.

Despite his findings in 1989, they were not released until 1997.

Dr. Burk examined a study that compared the 10 largest cities in the United States *with* fluoridation and the 10 largest cities that *do not* fluoridate their water. Following fluoridation, researchers discovered that deaths from cancer went up in as little as one year.

Researchers with Tulane University in New Orleans, Louisiana, discovered a revolutionary breakthrough that challenges the practice of fluoridation head on! It's a compound extracted from raw cacao called theobromine that strengthens tooth enamel.

If you live in a fluoridated community (and in the United States, you probably do), consider installing a reverse osmosis water filter. It will remove the fluoride as well as the majority of other nasty things found in tap water.

Natural Ways to Clean & Protect Your Teeth

One of the oldest and most effective ways to improve your oral health is using coconut oil. Ayurvedic practitioners have used this method for thousands of years and it still works today.

Discover the benefits of oil pulling to banish plaque, prevent disease, and protect your teeth! Listen to our podcast now!

Scientists have proven time and again that oral health directly impacts your overall wellness. Let's look at some natural methods for protecting your teeth and gums.

Non-Toxic Toothpaste Alternatives: Clay Toothpaste

Montmorillonite or Bentonite Clay is an all-natural compound that cleans and detoxifies your gums. The clay absorbs impurities and enhances gum repair. It has even been shown to remineralize cavities.

Caution! Do not let your clay toothpaste come into contact with metal. The negative charge of the ions in the clay will act as a magnet to the positive ions in the metal; they'll swap, and cause your clay to become semi-toxic.

You don't want that! Use a wooden spoon to mix your toothpaste and use a glass container for storage!

Ingredients
- 1½ tablespoons Bentonite Clay (see the resource section for what I use)
- 2 tablespoons distilled or purified water
- 1 tablespoon coconut oil melted
- ½ teaspoon sea salt (if you have sensitive teeth, skip the salt – but do not use table salt as a substitute)
- 2 teaspoons baking soda
- 5-10 drops of essential oil (clove, peppermint, lemon, orange, or grapefruit)
- Small glass container (do not use metal!)

Instructions
- Using a wooden or plastic spoon, mix water and clay to form a paste.
- Add all the other ingredients together and stir until thoroughly mixed.
- Store in a glass jar (do not use metal!).

Non-Toxic Toothpaste Alternatives: Baking Soda & Coconut Oil

Create a mixture of 2:1 (two parts baking soda to one part coconut oil). Dip your toothbrush in it and brush your teeth as you normally do.

For a minty fresh feeling, add a drop or two of peppermint, clove, or lemon essential oil to the mixture. I suggest storing your toothpaste in a non-porous glass container.

When choosing an essential you want to select pure unadulterated essentials oils. Most companies call their product "pure" when they are less than 30% and as little as 10% plant products. Check out Daily Superfood Love for excellent resources on choosing pure essential oils.

Non-Toxic Toothpaste Alternatives: Sea Salt

Dip your damp toothbrush in sea salt and brush away. If you're worried about abrasion, you can dissolve the salt in water first.

This will remove stubborn plaque, aid with healing if you suffer from ulcers, and essentially sterilize the inside of your mouth.

Common Toxic Offender #2 - Electromagnetic Radiation (EMR)

Cell phones are used by nearly all adults and teenagers in the developed world. Even children seem to carry them these days.

The electromagnetic radiation (EMR) they emit has dangerous long-term effects on the human body. EMR can alter and weaken cell membranes, increase the production of free radicals in the body, and even increase risk of cancers of the brain, nerves, neck, or head.

Dr. Devra Davis, an expert in this field, explains, "A cellphone is a two-way microwave radio. If people understood that they were holding a two-way microwave-radiating device next to their brain or next to their reproductive organs, they might think differently about it."

New research released at the annual American Society of Hypertension conference suggested that cell phones might need to be added to the list. Doctors from Guglielmo da Saliceto Hospital found that calls made on mobile phones acutely increased blood pressure readings from normal to as high as 129/82 during the course of the call.

Am I suggesting you give up your cell phone? Absolutely not! I rely on mine as you do. However, there are ways to minimize your exposure to EMR and still stay connected.

How to Reduce EMR Exposure from Cell Phones:

- Use a hands-free option to keep the cell phone away from your head as often as possible.

- Don't carry a cell phone in your pocket or tuck it (as we women tend to do) in your bra. Carry it at least 10mm (3/8") away from your body.

- Cases with metal components may change the RF performance of the cell phone in untested ways and have effects that have not been discovered.

- Meet with people face-to-face instead of on a device. It's a skill we're gradually losing in our modern world.

- Curb the frequency of your exposure. Ask yourself, "Do I really need to be texting, calling, watching, or listening on my cell phone all the time?"

Common Toxic Offender #3 - Bisphenol-A (BPA) and Bisphenol-S (BPS)

You've probably heard about BPA, one of the dangerous chemicals found in plastics. It's used in many water bottles, food containers, the lining of canned goods, and personal care product containers. BPS, a chemical that's lesser known and similar to BPA, is just as dangerous.

Both of these chemicals mimic *estrogen*.

They can interfere with the way cells respond to estrogen or even change cellular growth structure. Even small doses gradually become toxic. They are bio-accumulative, meaning that your body is unable to process them and they build up in your tissues.

- Choose glass jars over food packaged in cans, and fresh is always best.

- If you have a baby, throw out the plastic teething toys and choose those made of natural wood or fabric instead.

- BPS is found in thermal cash register paper, 87% of paper money, and 52% of recycled paper.

- It's even in the paper made for ultrasound machines.

Researchers have discovered BPS in the urine of a whopping **93% of Americans** they tested!

Common Toxic Offender #4 – Phthalates

Found in PVC flooring, padded play mats, and in many personal care toiletries including shampoo and cosmetics. Phthalates are endocrine disruptors and can cause developmental and hormonal damage.

It's critical to limit exposure.

- Replace vinyl shower curtains with fabric ones.

- Got *leftovers*? Skip the plastic wrap and store food in glass containers. Of course, you should never reheat food in plastic or Styrofoam packaging.

- Consider switching to natural brands of toiletries, shampoos, and toothpaste.

- Avoid synthetic fragrances found in perfumes, dryer sheets, laundry detergents, fabric softeners, or scented candles. Opt for natural cleaning products.

Find out how to clean naturally with citric acid and get the full scoop on making the switch to non-toxic disinfectants on Daily Superfood Love.

Implementing these simple changes can reduce your personal toxic exposure to everyday chemicals. Your cells and your home environment will feel brand new! Start today.

Revitalize Your Cells and Thank Spirulina

Take a deep breath. While you're doing that – thank spirulina. If not for these blue-green microalgae, you wouldn't have the air you're breathing.

It's one of the oldest life forms on Earth, and billions of years ago, it helped produce the oxygen that turned our planet into a place suitable for lifeforms like us.

After all this time, it's still working wonders.

Sometimes known as the original superfood, spirulina is one of the most nutrient-dense foods known to exist. It's rich in chlorophyll. Laboratory

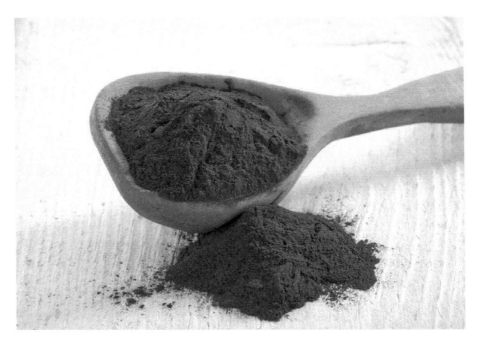

studies discovered you could literally survive and thrive on a diet of nothing but spirulina and water.

Admittedly, many would not find this to be the ideal diet! Instead, add it to your current healthy eating plan to gain access to the many benefits of spirulina.

What Makes Spirulina the Original Superfood?

All essential amino acids – present and accounted for.

Amino acids are small molecules that form proteins. They are crucial to every core process in your body. They build muscle, repair tissue, and maintain mood. Spirulina contains 65% protein and amino acids.

Burn more fat during exercise.

In a blind study, individuals taking spirulina supplements instead of a placebo decreased glucose oxidation by 11% – their bodies burned fat for energy.

Ramp up immunity!

Research has indicated that one of the benefits of spirulina is that it normalizes your body's T-cell count as well as boosting production of interferon. In essence, spirulina protects cell membranes so that invading viruses have difficulty attaching themselves to cells. This has proven effective against herpes, influenza, and HIV.

Every known antioxidant in one place.

Antioxidants are powerful cancer fighters, stopping and often reversing the damage caused by free radicals. When ranked on the Oxygen Radical Absorbance Capacity (ORAC) scale, which is a way of measuring a food's antioxidant concentration, spirulina is astounding.

It is the food richest in beta-carotene and contains ten mixed carotenoids. Blueberries, a high-antioxidant food, have an ORAC rating of 2400. Spirulina is rated at a staggering 25,300 on the ORAC scale!

Kick cancer's butt every step of the way.

Phycocyanin, a biliprotein in spirulina, inhibits cancer formation. One study conducted among tobacco chewers resulted in a total regression of precancerous mouth lesions among 45% of subjects given spirulina extracts for twelve months.

New research shows that spirulina binds with radioactive isotopes used during radiation and chemotherapy. Those isotopes kill healthy tissue as well as cancerous on their own. Spirulina offers healthy cells protection they wouldn't normally have.

Remove heavy metal out of your body – if not your playlist.

Heavy metals are everywhere in our toxic modern environment. Spirulina is high in chlorophyll, which helps removes toxins. It binds to them, enabling them to be flushed safely from your system.

Where do these metals come from? The air you breathe may contain cadmium and lead. The government allows an acceptable level of mercury in the fish you eat. Most deodorants contain aluminum. Essentially, heavy metal exposure can come from many sources you might not be aware of... and spirulina helps eliminate these from your body.

Keep the ticker strong and pumping for years longer.

Not only does spirulina contain high levels of omega-3s, it's been proven to reduce LDL "bad" cholesterol levels while elevating HDL "good" cholesterol levels in the body. This naturally lowers blood pressure and improves the health of your heart.

These are just a few of the many benefits you get from spirulina. This natural superfood has been safely used for thousands of years by many different cultures for everything from a food source to medicine.

When choosing spirulina, always opt for organic. It's not chocolate (by any means), so if you go for powdered spirulina, you can add 2 teaspoons to your daily smoothie. If you're sick of fighting an illness, take up to 2 tablespoons per day.

It doesn't have the best taste but when mixed into a morning shake, you can drink it down, recharge your cells, and get all the amazing health benefits without being overwhelmed by the taste.

If you prefer supplements, try *organic* spirulina capsules. Look for capsules that contain at least **450 mgs of spirulina** each. NASA studied it as a compact, easy to grow food for the astronauts on the International Space Station.

For those of us on the ground, spirulina is a recommended healthy addition to your daily life.

Your homework for today is to figure out what toxins you may have in your home. If you're like most of us, you'll mainly find them in your bathroom and kitchen. Make a list of changes needed to minimize your personal exposure every day.

Don't forget to drink your lemon water, do your poses, make your nutritious dinner, and give yourself a dry brush before your shower! Then climb into bed and visualize your ideal life.

Day 7
UNLEASH

TAKE BACK CONTROL OF YOUR LIFE & BECOME POWERFUL THROUGH EMOTIONAL RESILIENCE

You made it to the seventh day of Vivid Living! If you're here, I'm incredibly happy. It means you're committed to REAL change in your body, your mind, and your life.

I hope you're proud of the changes you're making, the steps you're taking, and the work you're willing to do to TRANSFORM your life and become physically and emotionally healthier.

Thank you for being a part of Vivid Living.

This last unit is a little emotional – no pun intended. Emotions are at the core of so many things in daily life. They dictate how you see yourself, how you interact with others, and how you view your worthiness of an amazing future.

Every day you're bombarded by actions or people that can flood your space with negativity in many different forms. Anger, selfishness, grief, hurt, anxiety, and even the lack of confidence from others can infect your day, your job, and your entire outlook.

You must become *emotionally resilient* – mentally build yourself up to deal with people or situations that can drain you one moment at a time if you don't guard against them.

Emotional resilience will help you effectively deal with negative or toxic people. You will no longer allow them to derail your day or stop you from achieving your personal mission in life.

The term 'emotional resilience' simply refers to one's ability to adapt to stressful situations in their life and continue to move forward.

Many people *covet* this trait! If you don't have it, I'm going to show you how to develop it. It's all about changing your mindset and your attitude. If you don't change what you are doing right now (or the way you've always done things), then you will always get the same result.

Ask yourself honestly, "*Is that really what you want?*"

There are people I know (and you likely know some as well) that always seem to roll with whatever life throws at them. They don't seem overly stressed out, they don't lose their composure if things go wrong, and they're probably a person many go to for advice.

That's a person with emotional resilience.

Let's talk about the Five Most Valuable Character Traits *emotionally resilient people possess – that you can learn to attain!*

They Know Their Boundaries

People who are emotionally resilient understand their boundaries in all areas. They understand that the stress and trauma they endure may be a part of their life, but it does not overtake their entire personality. Whenever they go through stressful situations, they don't take the situations personally and don't let their mood affect their manners.

They Keep Good Friends

Emotionally resilient people have very good friends. These people tend to seek out and surround themselves with other people who are emotionally resilient. For this reason, they also tend to *be* very good friends to have. They are supportive and know how to listen well.

They Are Self-Aware

Being blissfully unaware or going by the life motto "ignorance is bliss" may help you get through a hard day, but it won't be beneficial to yourself in the long term. Self-awareness and knowing your limits helps you to get in touch with what you need, what you don't need, and recognize when it's time to ask for help. Being self-aware can help keep your moods in check and even improve your health.

They Accept Things They Cannot Change

Pain and stress in your life are both horrible things to deal with no matter who you are. If you are emotionally resilient, you accept both and continue to move forward. Accepting the pain and stress that comes with life allows you to stop dwelling on your previous poor decisions or poor situations and allows you to keep learning, growing, and living.

They Are Willing to Be Silent

This can be one of the best skills to learn in life. Sometimes it's important to stay silent and passive in a stressful situation. Emotionally resilient people practice a concept known as mindfulness. This allows them to just be in the moment and not avoid their stressful situation.

Emotional resilience is something some people are born with but most who possess the trait have acquired it over the course of their lifetime. Experiences have taught them what constitutes a true "emergency" and anything less is calmly assessed and dealt with rationally.

I mentioned that many people covet this skill, this personality trait, because in our modern world, it's rather easy to hit the "panic" button.

A whisper of a new "deadly disease" can go globally viral – thanks to social media – within hours. Political, environmental, and personal health "Chicken Littles" are everywhere because they are easily heard.

Fortunately, the sky isn't usually falling.

If you recognize that you aren't as emotionally resilient as you'd like, or simply that you want to be the calm one in your life, you can attain the traits of emotional resilience with practice.

Here are Five Simple Ways to Cultivate Emotional Resilience *with regular practice and focus. I ask that you commit to working on just one of these exercises each day.*

Within weeks, developing these habits will change so much about how you see yourself and how you interact with others.

Make Connections

Emotionally resilient people have friends who are supportive, loving, and present in the ways that matter. In order to become emotionally resilient, make connections with *positive* and *encouraging* people who build you up and add to your quality of life.

Good relationships with your friends and family can help you cope with stress more effectively and reduce the amount of stress you feel from day to day.

Avoid Visualizing Your Crisis as Massive Problems

When you find yourself in a crisis or in a stressful situation, avoid making the problem even bigger than it is inside your head.

Instead, take a step back to determine if you are exaggerating an experience mentally or emotionally. If you are, reduce the size of the problem by making a list of the possible positive and negative outcomes.

Be prepared for the negatives but focus *only* on the positives!

Accept that Change Happens

Change happens, sometimes minute by minute. Unless you accept the fact that transitions occur, practice mindfulness when it comes to dealing with it, and surround yourself with like-minded people, change will always have a negative connotation in your life.

Not all change is bad and not all bad changes equal the end of life, as you know it. It's all about perspective.

Move Towards Your Goals

Everyone has goals emotionally resiliency depends heavily on always working towards those goals important to you. Take a step back and evaluate where you are right now. If you aren't currently doing things in your life that get you closer to your final goals, it's time to change your behaviors and attitude.

You must constantly be moving forward in order to build up your emotional resilience.

Build Up Your Self Confidence

Developing confidence in your ability and in your appearance builds resilience to anything life throws at you. When you are confident in your abilities and in yourself, you learn to trust your instincts.

Stop talking to yourself in a negative manner, and instead, build yourself up. Over time, you can boost your confidence levels and improve many aspects of your personal existence...including your emotional resilience.

Here are Four Life-Hacks to Crush It in Your Daily Life *that will build every aspect of resilience, including emotional, physical, mental, and social.* I love these action tips and I hope you will to.

This is today's **10-minute exercise to build resilience**! Get ready to unleash your true power and become emotionally and physically stronger right now!

You can do this!

- **Physical Resilience:** Stand with your arms up over your head for 60 seconds. Get up every hour and walk around for five minutes.

- **Mental Resilience:** Snap your fingers and count to 50 at the same time. Feel free to do it to your own internal rhythm!

- **Emotional Resilience:** Look at pictures or videos of baby animals for 60 seconds. No, seriously...kittens and puppies lift your mood (science proved it)!

- **Social Resilience:** Shake hands with someone once a day. Send a quick thank you email or tweet daily. Smile at service staff or co-workers – even if you don't really "feel" like smiling.

Emotionally resilient people are people who can bounce back when life throws a punch. No matter what, they are *survivors*, and are the envy of people struggling to cope.

You don't have to struggle anymore because you have the keys to unlocking this trait inside yourself.

YOU can now become a person who possesses emotional resiliency.

With these simple steps, you'll be able to rise up, meet life challenges, and create your own vivid life!

A FINAL MESSAGE...

Thank you for reading Vivid Living.

The fact that you're doing each day means you believe you're a worthy investment. You are the *best investment* you will ever make.

Congratulations! This book was written to fit into an active life – the crazy busy ones that most of us lead – so keep investing in you by continuing to practice it daily.

Remember...

1. Drink lemon water to replenish your cells and keep you hydrated.

2. Practice your poses for relaxation and power.

3. Give your body the fuel it needs in good food to live longer and stronger.

4. Visualize the life you want and actively take the steps to make it a reality.

5. Remove toxins from your body through dry brushing.

6. Guard against toxins in your environment and protect your body with spirulina.

7. Work to develop emotional resiliency.

Practice these actions and read Vivid Living as many times as you need to...until these actions are firm habits in your life.

Think of Vivid Living as your personal mini-action plan that will enable you to transform your mind, body, and spirit in ten minutes a day.

Live vividly today, tomorrow, and forever.

Vivid Living
10 MINUTE
WORKOUTS

10 MINUTE TOTAL BODY WORKOUTS TO BUILD ENDURANCE & STRENGTH

Set your timer for 10 minutes and go!

If you're sedentary, meaning you sit more than eight hours a day, or the most activity you get is walking to the coffee pot then I can help you. These bodyweight exercise routines were designed by our Daily Superfood Love resident fitness expert, certified personal trainer Dana Kavouklis, NASM-CPT.

"I created these powerful and easy to complete workouts to ease you into the daily routine of becoming more active without any of the fear associated, when you hear the words, "working out," said Dana.

If you already work out several times a week, then try the intermediate to advanced 10-minute total body workout.

Daily actions will become consistent habits. Don't think, worry, or over-analyze it. It's just 10 minutes. Set your timer and just do it! You can do these exercises every day. I guarantee within one week you'll notice an improvement in your stamina and you'll actually look forward to your strength-building routine.

Need more inspiration to get started?

Read Shayne's Journey from Sedentary to Energetic starting on page 113.

Ready to get started? Here's what we have in this 10-minute total body workout guide.

- Beginner Workout, Version 1

- Beginner Workout, Version 2

- Intermediate Workout, Version 1

- Intermediate Workout, Version 2

Starting on the next page, you'll be able to see examples and visuals of each exercise pose.

Vivid Tip: Download a **Tabata HIIT Timer** on your phone, laptop, or tablet. Set the work interval for 30 seconds, the rest interval for 10 seconds and the rounds (count) for 14 for the beginner's version one routine.

BEGINNERS

Version 1

Do these exercises in order and then repeat sequence for two sets in total.

Warm-up: 1 minute march in place

30 second squats

30 second wall push-ups

30 second modified jumping jacks (no jumping, step out and then back)

30 second alternating reverse lunges

30 second modified plank

30 second high knee pulls

30 second rest

Repeat sequence

Cool Down: End with one minute marching in place cool down. Extend your arms overhead and lower them (repeat) as you inhale through your nose, bring arms down as you exhale out the mouth.

Important Note: It's important to have a small cool down period, especially if you have poor circulation. The cool down helps prevent venous pooling after exercise. If you stop exercising abruptly and the blood pools in your lower body, it could lead to dizziness. Just march in place or walk for a few minutes and you will keep your circulation normal.

Version One Exercise Guide

Do these exercises in order and then repeat sequence for two sets in total
Warm-up: 1 minute march in place

1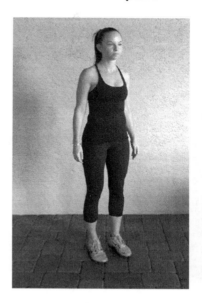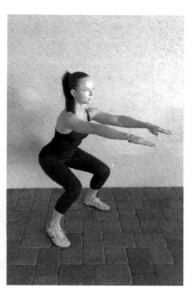

30 second squats

2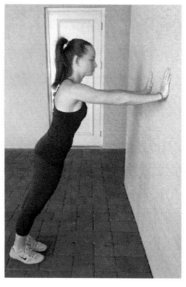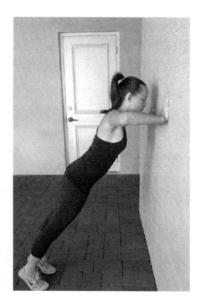

30 second wall push ups

3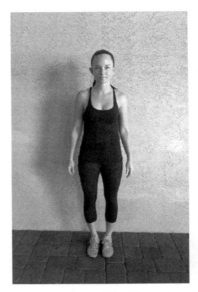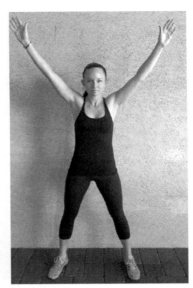

30 second modified jumping jacks (no jumping, step out, extend arms and then step back)

4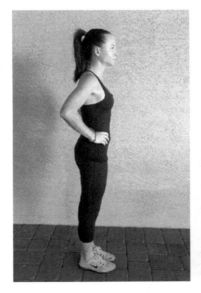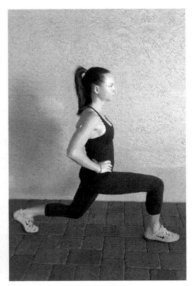

30 second alternating reverse lunges

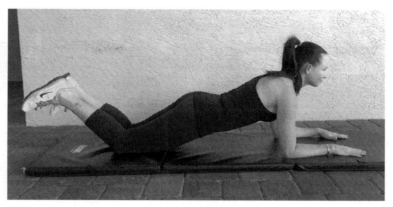

5

30 second modified plank (hold)

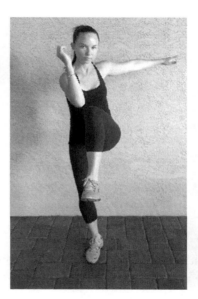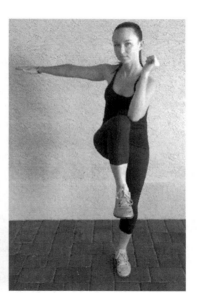

6

30 second high knee pulls

30 second rest

Repeat sequence

Cool Down: End with one minute marching in place cool down. Extend your arms up overhead and lower them (repeat) as you inhale through your nose, bring arms down as you exhale out the mouth.

BEGINNERS

Version 2

Do these exercises in order and then repeat sequence for two sets in total.

Warm-up: 1 minute march in place

10 squats

10 wall push-ups

30 second plank

1 minute high knee pulls or march

15 alternating reverse lunges

15 modified jumping jacks

30 second arm punches/jabs

1 minute high knee pulls or march

20 bridges

20 crunches

20 marching bridges (hips off floor, march feet bringing knees toward chest)

Repeat sequence

Cool Down: End with one minute marching in place cool down. Extend your arms overhead and lower them (repeat) as you inhale through your nose, bring arms down as you exhale out the mouth.

Important Note: It's important to have a small cool down period, especially if you have poor circulation. The cool down helps prevent venous pooling after exercise. If you stop exercising abruptly and the blood pools in your lower body, it could lead to dizziness. Just march in place or walk for a few minutes and you will keep your circulation normal.

Version Two Exercise Guide

Do these exercises in order and then repeat sequence for two sets in total.
Warm-up: 1 minute march in place

1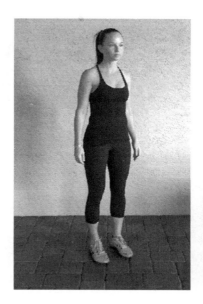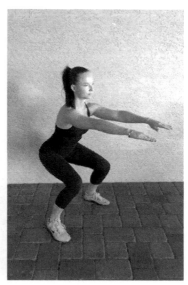

10 squats

2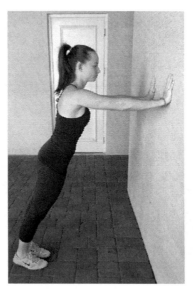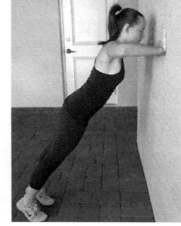

10 wall push-ups

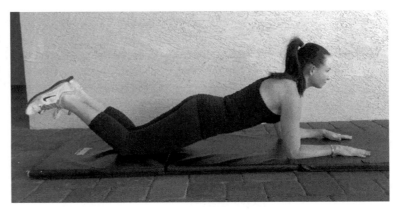

30 second plank

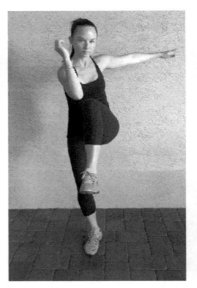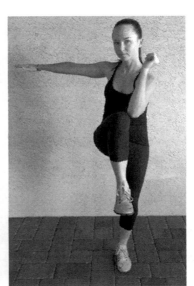

1 minute high knee pulls or march

5

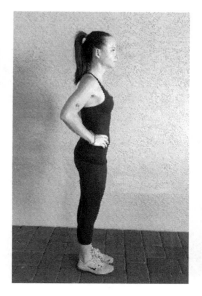 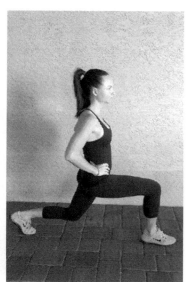

15 alternating reverse lunges

6

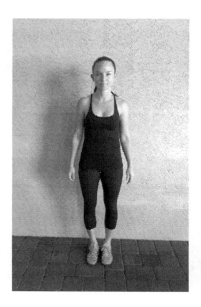 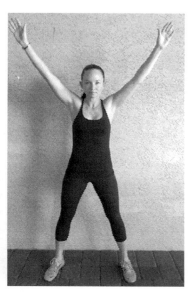

15 modified jumping jacks (step out and step back)

7

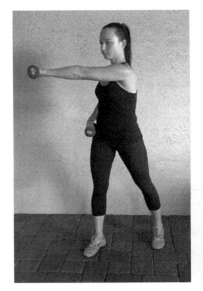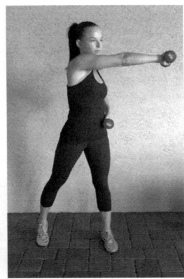

30 second arm punches/jabs (alternate arms)

8

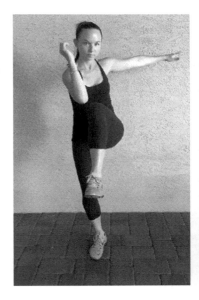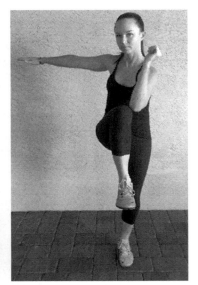

1 minute high knee pulls or march

9

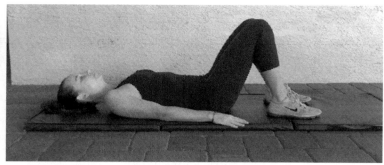

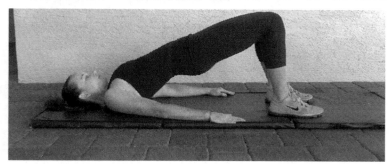

20 bridges

10

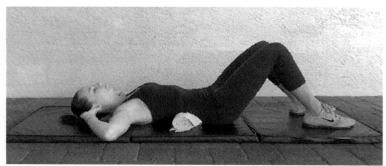

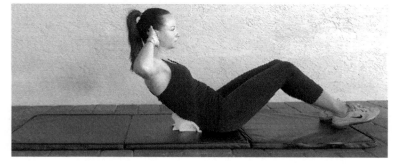

20 crunches

11

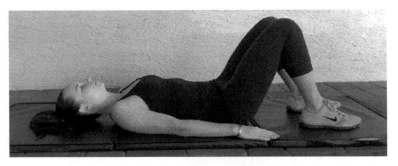

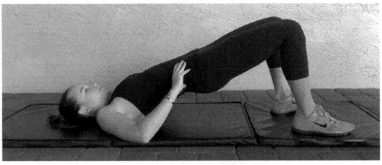

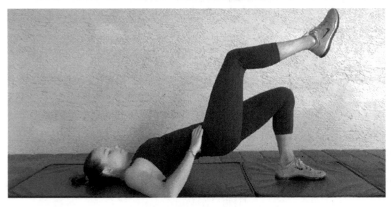

20 marching bridges...hips off floor, march feet bringing knees toward chest

30 second rest

Repeat sequence

Cool Down: End with one minute marching in place cool down. Extend your arms up overhead and lower them (repeat) as you inhale through your nose, bring arms down as you exhale out the mouth.

INTERMEDIATE TO ADVANCED

Version 1

Do these exercises in order and then repeat sequence for two sets in total.

Warm-up: 1 minute jog in place

30 second squats

30 second push-ups 30 second plank

30 second jumping jacks

30 second alternating reverse lunges with a front kick

30 second bicycle crunches

30 second rest

Repeat sequence

Cool Down: End with one minute marching in place cool down. Extend your arms overhead and lower them (repeat) as you inhale through your nose, bring arms down as you exhale out the mouth.

Important Note: It's important to have a small cool down period, especially if you have poor circulation. The cool down helps prevent venous pooling after exercise. If you stop exercising abruptly and the blood pools in your lower body, it could lead to dizziness. Just march in place or walk for a few minutes and you will keep your circulation normal.

Version One Exercise Guide

Do these exercises in order and then repeat sequence for two sets in total.
Warm-up: 1 minute jog in place

1

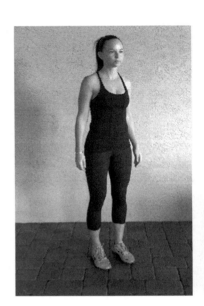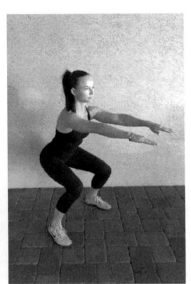

30 second squats

2

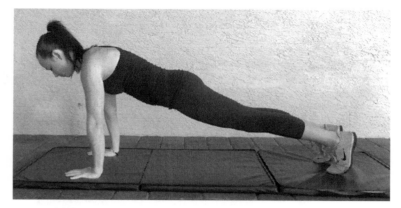

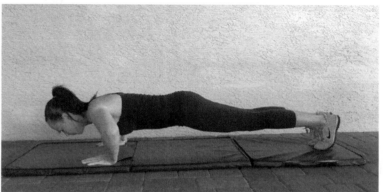

30 second push ups

3

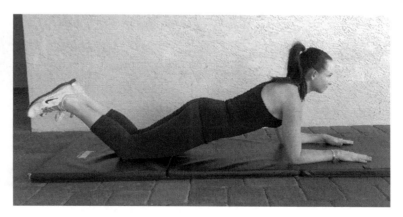

30 second plank

4

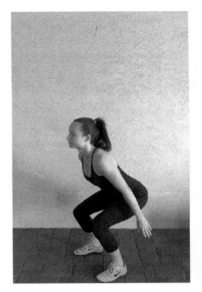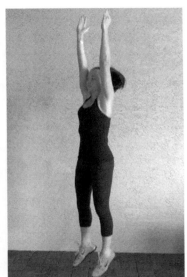

30 second jumping jacks

5

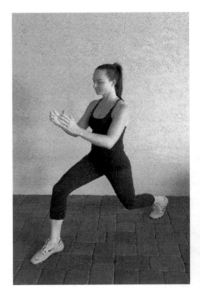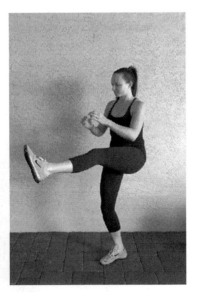

30 second alternating reverse lunges with a front kick

6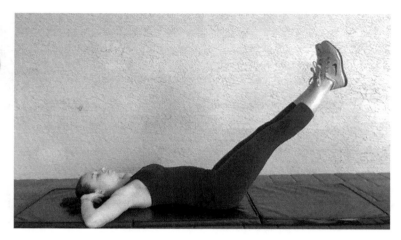

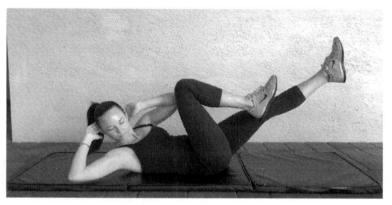

30 second bicycle crunches

30 second rest

Repeat sequence

Cool Down: End with one minute marching in place cool down. Extend your arms overhead and lower them (repeat) as you inhale through your nose, bring arms down as you exhale out the mouth.

INTERMEDIATE TO ADVANCED

Version 2

Do these 18 exercises in order and then repeat sequence for two sets in total.

Warm-up: 1 minute jog in place

10 squats
10 push ups
30 second plank
15 jump squats
15 push ups
30 second plank
20 squats w front kick 20 push ups
30 second plank
20 alternating front lunges
20 jumping jacks
30 second plank

15 reverse lunges w front kick
15 jumping jacks
30 second plank
10 plyo lunges
10 jumping jacks
30 second plank
1 minute march in place
Repeat sequence

Cool Down: End with one minute marching in place cool down. Extend your arms overhead and lower them (repeat) as you inhale through your nose, bring arms down as you exhale out the mouth.

Important Note: It's important to have a small cool down period, especially if you have poor circulation. The cool down helps prevent venous pooling after exercise. If you stop exercising abruptly and the blood pools in your lower body, it could lead to dizziness. Just march in place or walk for a few minutes and you will keep your circulation normal.

Version Two Exercise Guide

Do these exercises in order and then repeat sequence for two sets in total.
Warm-up: 1 minute jog in place

1

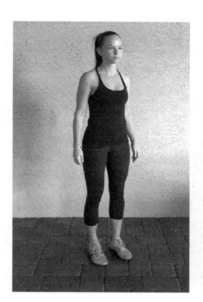 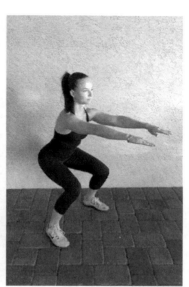

10 squats

2

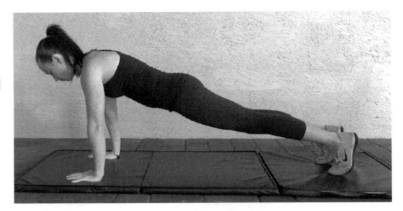

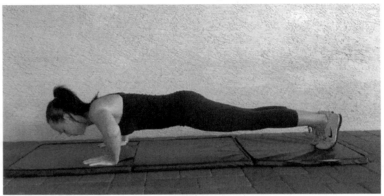

10 push ups

3

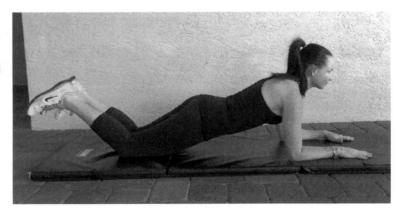

30 second plank

4

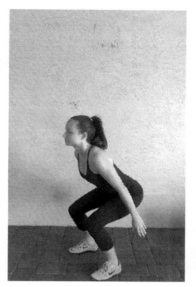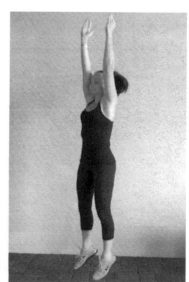

15 jump squats

5

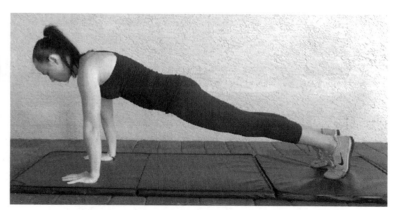
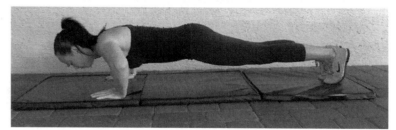

15 push ups

6

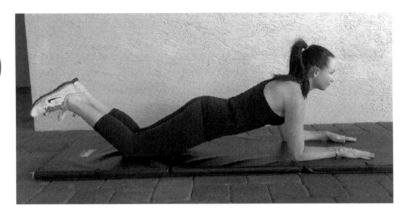

30 second plank

7

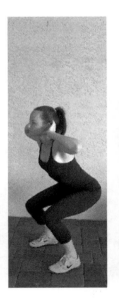 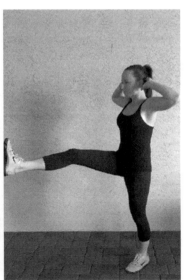

20 squats with front kick

8

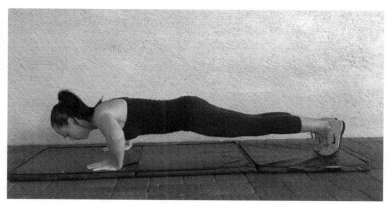

20 push ups

9

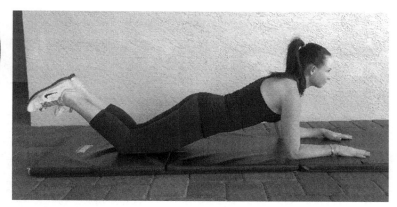

30 second plank

10

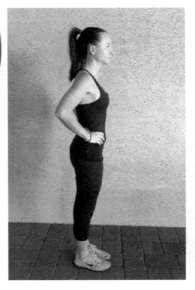
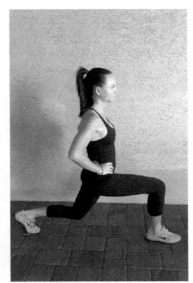

20 alternating front lunges

11

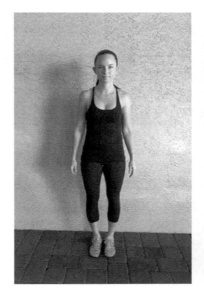
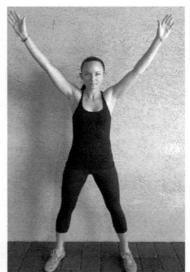

20 jumping jacks

12

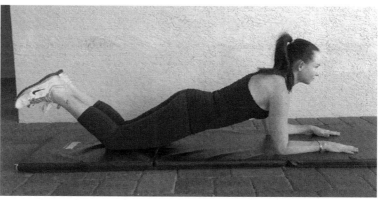

30 second plank

13

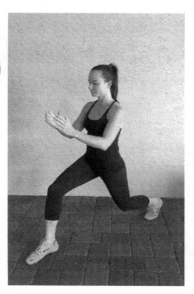
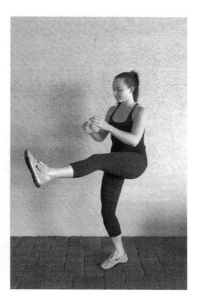

15 reverse lunges with front kick

14

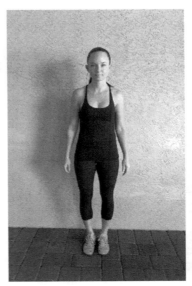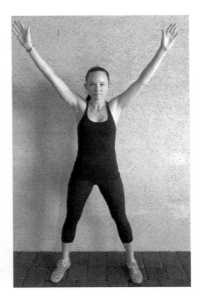

15 jumping jacks

15

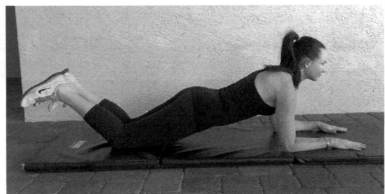

30 second plank

16

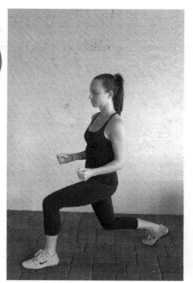
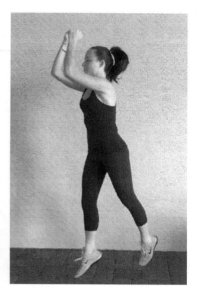
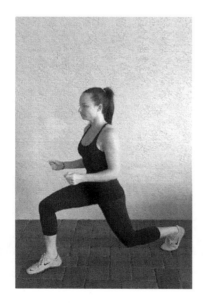

10 plyo lunges

17

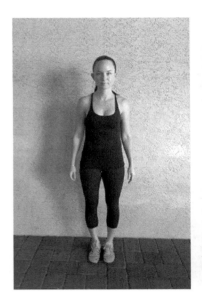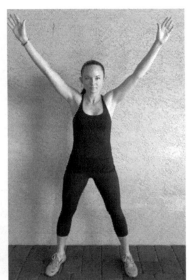

10 jumping jacks

18

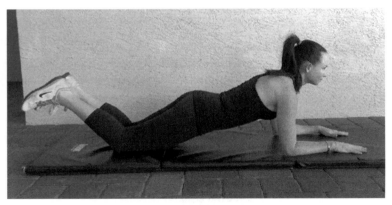

30 second plank

1 minute march in place

Repeat sequence

Cool Down: End with one minute marching in place cool down. Extend your arms overhead and lower them (repeat) as you inhale through your nose, bring arms down as you exhale out the mouth.

FROM SEDENTARY TO ENERGETIC

Shayne McClendon's One-Week Vivid Living Diary
Day 1: Exercise Challenge

I didn't die. No, I'm being serious. When my client asked me to test these exercises, I was a little bit scared. "I'm the most sedentary person I know," I explained. "That's why we want to test it on you," was the terrifying reply.

I mean...it's different when I say it (but she had a point).

As a writer, I sit in a chair all day. That is no exaggeration. The extent of my "exercise regimen" is going to get more coffee. A lot of people who would classify themselves as sedentary at least get a tiny amount of exercise walking from their house to their car and from their car to their office, I don't even get that much.

I pulled up the list, opened the stopwatch on my phone, and said a little prayer. And then...I did it. Two sets without passing out! I'm not saying they're easy but I can tell they work by the warming of my muscles and they can be done right here in my office, three feet from my desk.

The only trouble I had was the floor planking that made my dog incredibly happy and had to be replaced with another round of high knee pulls. The darling almost suffocated me because he thought it was time to play.

If I can survive the first day – and as I type this, I feel the effects of what I just did – so can you. Trust me on this. If someone like me can stop the world's deadlines and make it through ten minutes of low impact exercises...you can do it, too.

I think I could have done more than ten minutes but I'm glad that was the limit. My email was going off like crazy! For me, it's time to get back to work!

Until tomorrow,

Shayne

PS: Day One – Living Vividly. I normally drink my weight in coffee but this is changing a lot for me. However, despite the fact that I am running to the bathroom more than I did when I was 9 months pregnant, I have to say...I feel better.

Day 2: Exercise Challenge

Being sore already from house projects, I admit that I kind of dreaded doing my workout today. I woke up unable to feel my lower back.

To my shock, after two minutes of moving, I felt better than when I started. Am I still sore? Yup (I'm also 44, overweight, and move less than a snail) but not *as* sore (and there's definitely a difference). I have the feeling back in that area right above my butt – the "upper butt" muscles that were pretty much numb (except for an occasional fiery twinge that was rather unpleasant) this morning.

I can also touch my toes (almost) again. I thought we were broken up for good this time. Turns out, they missed me, we're talking, I think it's going to be okay.

It was easier today and I only had to remind myself of the next exercise once – I stopped the clock to double check. Clearly, I need to print it out... duh.

I'm finished, typing this, and realize that I'm super proud of me right now. Something else I've noticed in the first two days: the world didn't end! It's a shocker to discover that taking ten minutes to do something personal didn't cause a catastrophic event from which I will never recover.

This was news to me. I tend to be a Nervous Nelly.

So! My takeaway is A) it's getting easier, B) I'm proud of myself for doing it, and C) the sky did not fall down around me.

Though I get a little more winded than most people will, I'm honestly looking forward to doing Day Three. Who's got this??? THIS GIRL!!!

Until tomorrow,

Shayne

PS: Day Two – Living Vividly. I'd forgotten how to take a few minutes to just breathe. Add to that the fact that I don't move around much and day two was ideal for my situation. At first, it felt strange to do nothing at all for several minutes. I was so glad I did.

Day 3: Exercise Challenge

I won't lie to you...the hardest part about doing these exercises is *not* the exercises. It's stopping all my crazy daily world and actually allowing myself the ten minutes to do them. Isn't it funny how we have so much time for ridiculous crap but can't give ourselves TEN minutes?

When I was first approached to be the test subject, I was worried about the exercises. I figured my old and out of shape self would keel over in the process. Each day, those get easier.

The hard part is letting myself walk away from work/family long enough to do them.

Today, I was able to finish the exercises in just over 9 minutes. Because of that, I did an extra 30 seconds of marching in place. I was proud of myself and I think it's a sign of progress.

My ability to put myself in the top priority slot? I'm still working on that.

Until tomorrow,
Shayne

PS: Day Three – Living Vividly. This is the easiest part for me so far. Putting new habits in place is harder than expanding good habits you already have so with a couple of tweaks to what I was doing, I feel like I have this Vivid Living step on lock!

Day 5: Exercise Challenge

I ended up skipping a day and it made me so angry because I'd been on track for three days in a row! Ugh! I was so disappointed in myself.

Today, I woke up extra early so I could do the exercises before the pressure of my daily task list fell on me. I found that doing them first actually helped. I felt amazing that I got them done and I was energized to face the rest of my day. My healthy shake hit the spot and then I allowed myself to sip coffee for three hours before switching to the better habit I'm working hard to form.

I have to be nicer to myself and not beat myself up. I think what made all the difference (from a hundred other "systems" I've tried to put in place) is that I got back on track. Maybe it was because I was testing these for a client or maybe I realized how good I was starting to feel.

Either way, I did them and I added almost 40 seconds of against the wall pushups to give myself a little extra for missing yesterday. This series of exercises aren't high impact. I might eventually do them first thing in the morning and again before I shower for bed.

Until tomorrow, Shayne

PS: The Day Four – Living Vividly assignment. Wow. Just...wow. That "homework" was ideal for me. This helped me with so many things I've been struggling to overcome. I hope you love it as much as I do!

Day 6: Exercise Challenge:

Just to test it, I did my exercises twice, in the morning and again at night. I might have to cut them in half if I do them so close to bedtime. I needed to sleep but my mind was racing as if I'd had a couple of energy drinks.

I tend to be a night owl so...yeah, that's a bad idea. Another thing I decided was to try Day Two in Vivid Living instead. Duh! That was suggested but I've been doing it in the morning.

Part of this whole "change your life" thing for me is remembering that I can make it flexible, I can move it around, and I can alter it to fit me like a glove.

I've been in some very bad habits for a long time. I went through each day "reacting" to my life instead of "charting" it.

I think I'll change up a couple of these ideas and place them like oasis spots through my day. It will break things up and help me recharge.

This is working. I feel amazing. I want to stick to it...I deserve it.

Until tomorrow,
Shayne

PS: Day Five – Living Vividly assignment...before I did it, I made a face. I thought it was silly and no way could it work (blah, blah, blah). All I can tell you now is that I stand corrected. It is so weird and yet afterward, made so much sense. Shivers all over and I felt as if I could feel my skin "perking" up. Do it and tell me your first reaction!

Day 7: Exercise Challenge (and Overview)

One series of the exercises in the morning (they took me a solid 9 so I added some squats – my legs never move), all my "Living Vividly" habits scattered on the odd hours, a break at lunch to do a half-set of the exercises, food, some downtime with my daughter, and then my "wind down" 20 minutes before shower and bed.

I slept like a rock and woke up ready to conquer the world.

Here are my overall thoughts about this system:

At the end of the last day on the challenge, I realized (as I was doing my Living Vividly homework) that I have followed a solid week of tasks designed to make me think about myself...that forced me to remember that my health and wellbeing are as important as the health and wellbeing of the people I love.

I can't tell you how proud that makes me. My test for the client is finished but as I make a couple of important "to do" lists, I recognize that these are pretty easy to incorporate in my life as it is right now...no matter how crazy busy I am and how little "spare" time I have.

I want to feel good. I want to take an active role in my own life. I want to be healthy, I want to live a long time, and I want the energy to accomplish the ridiculous amounts of things I load on my daily agenda.

These techniques are simple and if I can do them – you can do them.

I'm out of shape, I'm distracted, and I have a lot of demands for my time and attention (workwise and personally). I estimate that I actually devoted 15 minutes of my day to Vivid Living...factoring a few things in the place of what I used to do. New, never done before, about 15 minutes.

I feel refreshed and recharged. I feel as if I've exhaled fully for the first time in a long time. Now, a deep breath in...

Choose to live a vivid life,
Shayne

Made in the USA
Charleston, SC
09 January 2017